Scientific Advances Regarding:

Sugar,
Salt, & FAT

SECOND EDITION

by Gina Willett, R.D., Ph.D.

Biomed General
Concord, California
© 2015

Scientific Advances Regarding:
Sugar, Salt, & Fat 2nd edition

First edition: Sugar, Salt, & Fat / 2011
Second edition: Scientific Advances Regarding: Sugar, Salt, & Fat / 2015

ISBN: 978-1-893549-23-4

Biomed General
P.O. Box 5727
Concord, CA 94524-0727
USA

925.288.3500 *main*
925.680.1201 *fax*
info@biocorp.com

Author
Gina Willett, Ph.D., R.D.

Editor
Holly Stevens

Cover Art and Layout
Nancy Loquellano

About Biomed General

Biomed General is an organization that provides health care professionals with the latest scientific and clinical information. Biomed's live seminars and home-study courses are designed to help health professionals provide better care for their patients. Biomed General operates nationwide in the United States as well as internationally.

Biomed General

P.O. Box 5757
Concord, CA 94524-0757
USA

925-288-3500 *(main)*
925-680-1201 *(fax)*
info@biocorp.com

About The Author

Dr. Gina Willett (Ph.D., R.D.) is a nationally known speaker in the areas of nutrition, health, and wellness. She has a doctoral degree in nutrition and a master's degree in preventive medicine from the University of Wisconsin, Madison. She also has a master's degree in health education from the University of Oklahoma, Oklahoma City. Dr. Willett has worked as a Clinical Dietitian and Health Promotion Coordinator for the United States Air Force, as well as an Assistant Professor at the University of Richmond in Virginia. She now presents seminars to health professionals across the country and develops continuing-education courses.

Table of Contents

List of Figures

List of Tables

Chapter 1

Why Can't We Eat Just One?

W e've all heard that famous advertising campaign that reads, "Bet you can't eat just one." And, chances are, they could be right. Today's grocery stores and fast-food restaurants offer a tremendous variety of extremely palatable foods that are so tasty, many people simply can't resist eating them—and often overindulge as a result. But what is it that makes foods so darn tasty? What is it about *certain* foods that give them such power over us? As we will see in this book, the allure of most hyperpalatable foods can be summarized in three words: *sugar, salt,* and *fat.*

You can think of sugar, salt, and fat as powerful forces of nature, found in *unnaturally* potent concentrations

1

in many of today's processed and packaged foods. These three ingredients don't simply provide pleasure (i.e., make our brain's "Twinkie" circuits light up), they also serve are miracle ingredients that are heavily exploited by food manufacturers (the "Food Giants"). As we will see, sugar, salt, and fat are key factors that are contributing to the success of our $1 trillion food industry and, in the process, are fueling America's obesity epidemic, putting millions, including our kids, at risk for heart disease, diabetes, and other chronic diseases.

Pulitzer-Prize-winning journalist Michael Moss[1] has taken an inside look at some of the biggest players in our food industry, exploring how they meticulously engineer foods, tweaking the ratios of sugar, salt, and fat, to optimize the pleasure. Executives and food scientists employed by the Food Giants want to create the biggest craving, so as to keep their "heavy users" using, and to hook new consumers, especially children, on their products (products Michael Pollan[2] refers as: "edible food-like substances"). And, as we'll see, they accomplish their goal with an approach similar to the way the cigarette industry hooked smokers on nicotine. With billions of advertising and marketing dollars, the food industry entices us with products laden with sugar, salt, and fat so as to foster an intense desire for hyper-processed foods, or what Dr. David A Kessler, former Food and Drug Administration director, refers to as a state of *conditioned hypereating*.[3]

So, what can we do to protect ourselves against the pull of poor-quality foods (or edible food-like substances)? The first step is to improve our nutritional literacy. By educating ourselves, our patients, clients, coworkers, families, friends, schools, neighbors, churches, and communities, we can make better choices—choices that ensure our physical and mental health. Knowledge impacts our buying practices. Voting *with your wallets and your forks* will, ultimately, shape the behavior of the Food Giants. It will influence the products they sell, and make them more accountable for the physical and social costs of their actions. This book is designed to arm you with knowledge and to motivate you to make the choices that will enable you to reclaim both your physical and mental health. Let's start with the basics.

What Motivates Us to Eat?

Metabolic & Hedonic (Pleasurable) Drives that Control Appetite: Who's Really the Boss?

Why do we succumb to the pull of food? Why is that we see people who can manage successful careers, maybe run a business and manage their finances and families...but they just seem totally powerless over that darn little chocolate in the shiny wrapper. How can inanimate objects, such as M&Ms®, cookies, and potato chips, acquire so much power over us...that they thoroughly dominate our attention...and make us feel as though we are spinning out of control?

Eating may seem basic, but the whole process, from feeling hungry to finally pushing ourselves away from the table, is controlled by an elaborate, and still largely mysterious, circuitry occurring between the body and the brain. There are two key systems that work hand-in-hand to influence our drive to eat *(see **Figure 1**)*.[4] The first is called the *homeostatic*

Figure 1. *Human homeostatic and hedonic systems*

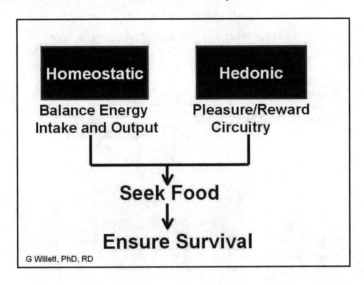

(or *metabolic*) system. The wisdom of the body is maintained through a feedback system known as *homeostasis*. Just like variables such as temperature, blood pressure, or blood sugar, which the body tries to maintain within relatively narrow ranges, our energy or fat stores are also *supposed to be* regulated by a homeostatic process that is designed to balance energy (or calorie) intake with energy expenditure. The "command center" of the homeostatic system is the *hypothalamus,* located at the base of the brain. The hypothalamus continually receives signals from the periphery (nutrients in the blood and hormones

Figure 2. *The homeostatic system*

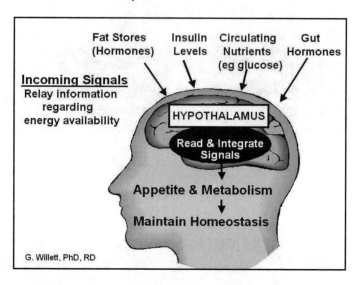

derived from the gastrointestinal tract, fat tissue, etc.), which inform the brain about the availability of fuel sources *(see **Figure 2**)*. The hypothalamus must accurately read and integrate these incoming signals, so as to regulate appetite and maintain a sufficient fuel supply so that we can achieve homeostasis, or balance in the body.[4] However, while this homeostatic system is vital for our survival, it does not work *alone*. If it did, there might not be sufficient drive to encourage us to eat and to store enough calories to protect us against starvation or famine. That drive is provided by the second system, the *hedonic* (or pleasure-reward) system.

Let's face it: In our modern world, we no longer eat *only* when we are metabolically hungry. In fact, many of us eat in complete absence of hunger (or metabolic need), and in spite of large fat reserves. And when we make food choices, it may not be the nutritional value of a food that's on the forefront of our minds. Instead, it's the taste, the flavor, the sensory satisfaction. This kind of eating is referred to as hedonic or *non-homeostatic* eating. It's a drive to seek that which gives us pleasure—a drive that is controlled by our *hedonic system*, a very complicated system that is influenced by a number of cognitive, reward, and emotional factors.[5]

Contrary to popular opinion, the hedonic system isn't just there for fun!!! On the contrary: Our brains are *hardwired* to respond and seek rewards that are essential for our survival. The hedonic system was designed, or evolved (depending on your perspective), to guide us to eat, rather than waste away, and to encourage us to procreate so that our genetic lineage doesn't die out. In the time of our ancestors, those with the strongest desire to seek food and to procreate were the ones who were most successful in surviving and passing on their genes. And, even though it's been several hundred generations, the fact of the matter is, we're still carrying around pretty much the same equipment upstairs as our distant ancestors did.

The hedonic system is housed in what is referred to as the *mesolimbic system* of the brain, earlier referred to as the Twinkie circuitry of the brain. That's because neuroimaging studies of this pleasure circuitry have shown that all it takes is one smell, sight, or taste of palatable food, and, instantly, a series of sensory, metabolic, and neurochemical fireworks go off in the brain that make us want that food, or *more* of that food. More specifically, palatable food induces a very potent release of a brain chemical called *dopamine*. Dopamine is the chemical in your brain chemical that makes you say "aah." Think of it as a chemical version of a "high-five," central to virtually anything that feels good, whether it's expensive chocolate, romantic flirtation, enjoyable music, or drugs. This pleasure chemical is released into an area of the brain called the *nucleus accumbens* (a.k.a. the *ventral striatum*), thought to be the epi-center of this pleasure circuit or the hedonic "hot spot," even though it measures only about the size of the head of a pin. If you stimulate this hot spot it magnifies the pleasure. It's like adding an extra layer of pleasure gloss. In general, the greater the release of dopamine, the more intense the experience of pleasure. The more intense the experience of pleasure, the greater the trigger, or the urge. So you feel pulled, like steel to a magnet (or a dieter to a chocolate cupcake!).

The release of dopamine is believed to coordinate many aspects of food reward, including increased arousal and attention, psychomotor activation, and conditioned learning (i.e., remembering food-associated stimuli).[3,6] Such a response was important for our ancestors, when palatable food was scarce. But our problem today is quite the opposite. We are constantly bombarded by highly palatable foods, such that the part of our brain that governs our rational responses (you know, the part that says to you

"you really need to get some sleep, not have another pint of Rocky Road ice cream"), can get overridden. We just can't resist. For some of us, the inner battle between our rational side and our Twinkie circuit is fought dozens of times a day.

Highly Palatable Foods "Rewire" the Brain, Making Us Want More (and More)....and That Can Get Us in Trouble

Normally, the homeostatic and hedonic systems are complementary *(see Figure 1)*—they work hand-in-hand, like a finely tuned system. But what's going wrong for some of us, that it may seem more like a beast in need of taming? Well, the core problem is that these systems were not designed to handle the kind of *obesogenic* food environment we face today. We have highly palatable, but poor quality food that is readily available, and heavily advertised and marketed... to the point that we're literally being bombarded by hyperpalatable foods. Today, our diets are essentially supercharging our reward systems! As a result, for many of us, our hedonic system is *overriding* our homeostatic controls. The hedonic system is taking the reins. It's running the show! Thus, we end up eating more often for pleasure than actual biological need. In other words, the hyperpalatability of our current food supply is undermining our normal satiety signals, stimulating the drive to eat even when there is no physiological need for food.[3,7] It is overpowering the brain's ability to tell us when to stop eating. And, in some cases, the more someone eats, the more he or she wants. An excessive hedonic drive can often represent an attempt to try to feel better, to relieve stress, to escape, or to seek comfort. That may explain why hedonic eating has many parallels with addiction mechanisms.

> The hyperpalatability of our current food supply is undermining our normal satiety signals, stimulating the drive to eat even when there is no physiological need for food.

The reinforcing properties of food. Considerable evidence in animals and humans supports the theory that both drugs of abuse and the consumption of highly palatable foods (i.e., those high in fat and sugar) converge on a shared pathway in the mesolimbic system to motivate behavior.[4] In other words, modern-day foods appear to have reinforcing abilities similar to alcohol or other drugs of abuse.[8] Once ingested, narcotics and food—especially food that is high in sugar, salt, and fat—race along the same pathways, using the exact same neurological circuitry to reach the brain's pleasure centers. Imaging studies have clearly demonstrated that highly palatable foods can light up the same pleasure centers in our brains that, for example, cocaine does, sending the message. "Eat more, eat more!"

Michael Moss[1] describes how, years ago, Unilever, makers of brands such as Breyers'® and Ben & Jerry's, put graduate students in an MRI machine and then scanned their brains as an assistant spooned vanilla ice cream into their mouths. What happened? Their brains' pleasure centers lit up instantly and brightly too, providing, for the first time ever, sound scientific evidence that ice cream really does make you happy… or, at least, give you pleasure. Unilever released the results, generating a flurry of publicity with their slogan, "Ice Cream Makes You Happy—It's Official!"

The link between food and drugs can be seen in many studies. One research project used a positron emission tomography brain scan to compare the brain structures of a cocaine addict to that of a food addict. When cocaine addicts observed a video of someone snorting cocaine, the reward region of their brains surged with dopamine.[9] However, in comparison, when they exposed non-drug addicts to images of a delicious cheeseburger, they observed the same surges of dopamine in the exact same parts of the brain. Another study[10] showed that the compulsion for binge eaters to overindulge in high-fat, high-sugar foods such as chocolate chip cookies, can actually be suppressed by the same drug, called naloxone, which is prescribed to block and counter the effects of heroin.

The concept of food addiction. Now, it's one thing to enjoy food and to experience a pleasurable dopamine brain reward when you consume it, but it's quite another to be so drawn to that food that you feel as though you are losing control. This phenomenon has been referred to as "food addiction" in both the lay media and the scientific literature.[11,12] And while for years experts scoffed at the notion that you could be hooked on chocolate or chips, we now have some rather striking scientific evidence that supports this concept. Of course no one is suggesting that an addiction to food could be as strong as an addiction to cocaine or heroin. After all, we don't see too many people robbing convenience stores to get their hands on Twinkies! But it is clear that the neurocircuitry is similar; it overlaps.

In May of 2013, the American Psychiatric Association (APA) unveiled its updated *Diagnostic and Statistical Manual of Mental Disorders, Fifth Edition (DSM-5)*.[13] While it included Binge Eating Disorder as a diagnostic category, it did not directly address the concept of food addiction. However, in the introduction to the "Feeding and Eating Disorders" section of the *DSM-5*, it stated:

> Some individuals with disorders described in this chapter report eating-related symptoms resembling those typically endorsed by individuals with substance-use disorders, such as strong craving and patterns of compulsive use. The resemblance

may reflect the involvement of the same neural systems, including those implicated in regulatory self-control and reward in both groups of disorders. However, the relative contributions of shared and distinct factors in the development and perpetuation of eating and substance use disorder remain insufficiently understood.

Despite the lack of a specific designation in the *DSM-5*, many experts are now defining "food addiction" in relation to the definition of substance abuse, using the Yale Food Addiction Scale.[14]

It appears that some individuals may be at greater risk for addiction, perhaps because they have heightened reactivity or responsivity to food cues. For example, it has been shown that the brain reward regions of individuals with higher food addiction scores tend to show greater brain activation in response to those cues that signal the impending delivery of desirable food (e.g., chocolate milkshake).[15] Based on this type of information, researchers have concluded that certain individuals are more likely to react or respond to food cues, and that the anticipation of a reward, when a cue is noticed, could contribute to compulsive eating behavior. But that heightened brain response may not be limited just to food. In a prospective brain imaging study (using magnetic resonance imaging; MRI), it was demonstrated that adolescents with elevated responsivity to rewarding stimuli were also at increased risk for the initiation and escalation of drug and alcohol abuse as well.[16] These findings shed important new light on the complex mechanisms that explain why some people are more prone to addictive behaviors, such as substance abuse and, perhaps, overeating, than others. But greater reactivity might be only part of the story. It's one thing to be attracted to a food cue; it's quite another to completely lose control and binge on that food. Perhaps part of the problem may be that, while the brain's reward centers light up in anticipation of a food reward (i.e., you get an *anticipatory* reward), it appears that for some people the actual consumption of food doesn't necessarily provide the expected reward (i.e., there's a lack of a *consummatory* reward). And, some

> Chronic exposure to a poor diet is capable of weakening our braking systems, causing us to lose control of our ability to regulate food consumption.

research suggests that it could be the excess quantities of poor quality food *itself* that are to blame for this blunted response.

If we continue to consume a poor quality, hyperpalatable diet, then, over time, this dietary pattern could cause changes or alterations in neuronal circuitry that make it difficult for us to control our food intake.[17] Research shows that both obese/overeaters and drug-addicted individuals suffer from impairments in dopaminergic pathways.[18] Scientific evidence suggests that *repeated exposure* to large amounts of palatable foods can *alter* the brain in ways similar to drugs of abuse, essentially "rewiring" the brain to promote compulsive overeating and loss of control.[6,19,20] The reason? Both refined foods and recreational drugs *overload* the brain's dopamine-pleasure center. Over time, this decreased sensitivity (*downregulation,* or erosion of the reward system) may prompt an individual to eat compulsively in an attempt to *regain* a sense of reward, at least temporarily. This would suggest that the more you do things that are *unnaturally* rewarding, the less reward you get from them. In this regard, compulsive overeating produces neuroadaptations that resemble drug addiction—adaptations that alter the motivation to obtain either type of reward—food *or* drugs.[6,21] In essence, chronic exposure to a poor diet is capable of weakening our braking systems, causing us to lose control of our ability to regulate food consumption.

> The more you do things that are **unnaturally** rewarding, the less reward you get from them.

One of the *DSM-5* criteria[13] for Substance Use Disorder is **tolerance**, which is defined by either of the following: (1) a need for markedly increased amounts of the substance to achieve intoxication or desired effect; or (2) a markedly diminished effect with continued use of the same amount of the substance. When animals are given intermittent access to sugar water, they will consume more and more sugar water until they are essentially bingeing on sugar water—a pattern of tolerance. For humans, tolerance might be reflected by statements such as, "If I tell myself I will only eat one cookie, then that leads to another and another until I make myself stop at five or six. I used to be able to eat only one or two." Or, "When I used to buy groceries, I would take them home, eat a snack and go on with my day. Now I buy groceries and I eat all day long until I have gone through half of what I bought."[22] There is a drive to consume larger and larger amounts of particular foods, or a substance (edible food-like substance) to get the same "hit." From a scientific perspective, tolerance is thought to reflect reduced sensitivity to dopamine by post-synaptic neurons in the nucleus accumbens, the hedonic hotspot.[23]

A second criterion for Substance Use Disorder[13] is **withdrawal**, which is manifested by either of the following: (1) the characteristic withdrawal syndrome for the substance; or (2) the same (or closely related) substance is taken to relieve or avoid withdrawal symptoms. Interestingly, animal models indicate that repeated, intermittent access to palatable foods, such as sugar water, can lead to both emotional and somatic signs of withdrawal when the food is no longer available.[24] Research has demonstrated the emergence of depressive-like behavior when animals are forced to withdraw from their highly palatable food, and these animals will quickly return to that food, as soon as possible, in order to relieve the withdrawal-induced negative emotional state.[25] However, while you might typically think that withdrawal symptoms are mostly *psychological* manifestations, such as seen with smoking cessation, in which the psychological withdrawal from cigarettes is often more prominent than the physical withdrawal, animal models demonstrate that a *physical* withdrawal phenomenon can also take place with regard to food. The animals become anxious, their teeth start to chatter, their heads shake, and they show a tremor in their forepaws. In humans, such a response may be manifested by statements such as, "Cutting down on starches makes me shaky." Or, "I eat sugar-filled foods so I am not as tired and/or depressed."[22] Interestingly, when animals are taken off of sugar water, but then given access to alcohol, they will increase their alcohol intake, suggesting that intermittent access to sugar can act as a gateway to, or cross-sensitize with, alcohol use. Intermittent access to sugar has also been shown to cross-sensitize with amphetamines, as well as cocaine, in animal models, thus suggesting that food-related dependence may influence susceptibility to drug addiction.[26,27] High fat diets have also been shown to stimulate dopamine release in the nucleus accumbens. However, the same type of withdrawal symptoms have *not* been observed when animals were forced to abstain from fat, or were treated with naloxone.[23,26]

The role of genetic factors. While it's clear that a poor quality diet may downregulate our reward systems to promote overeating *(see **Figure 3**)*, there is evidence that some overeaters may *start out* with weaker or blunted reward circuitry (perhaps due to genetic differences in the dopamine system, e.g., a decreased number of dopamine receptors).[28] As a result, they may be driven to try to increase their dopamine response, possibly through the use of illicit drugs or, more commonly, through compulsive overeating. Thus, these individuals are eating more, or overcompensating, in an attempt to achieve a greater dopamine reward. The more blunted their

Figure 3. *Overeating and blunted reward circuitry: Interaction between nature and nurture*

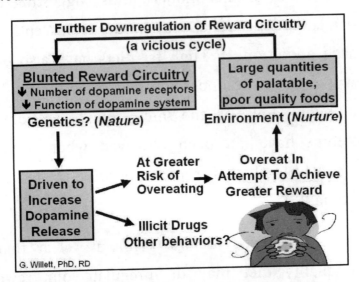

dopamine response, the more likely they are to overeat. But it may not just be food; they could be vulnerable to *anything* that fulfills the missing sense of dopamine reward they are seeking. So, there may be one family member who is hooked on refined foods, another hooked on wine, another drugs, another compulsive shopping, another video gaming, etc. Or, they may have multiple addictions or compulsions. This may explain the phenomenon of replacing food addiction with other dependencies, such as alcohol, after bariatric surgery—a phenomenon now termed "addiction transfer."[29]

Thus, a person with weaker reward circuitry may *continue* to eat in an attempt to capture a greater sense of reward. But here's the problem: They're probably not driven to eat large quantities of broccoli; they're driven to eat more of the highly palatable foods to achieve the greatest dopamine release. The more poor quality foods they consume, the greater the down regulation of the dopamine reward system.[28] And the more the dopamine response is dulled, the greater the drive to raise dopamine levels, and so on, and so on…until it becomes a vicious cycle *(Figure 3)*. This is what is meant by saying that their brains are being "rewired."

So, what came first, nature or nurture? Both drug abuse and obesity/overeating are associated with alterations or decreased sensitivity of the dopamine reward system. But the direction of the causality is not known. Did a pre-existing risk factor (i.e, genetics, or "nature") disturb the system or blunt the reward circuitry, thus predisposing an individual to abuse drugs or food? We know that both obesity and addiction run in families. And, if that is the case, it certainly puts to rest the notion that overeaters simply lack willpower. What they may be missing instead is a normally functioning dopamine reward system.[28] Or, could it be that the decreased sensitivity of the dopamine reward system is the result of repeated over-stimulation of the system (i.e., the result of the environment, or "nurture")? Animal research suggests that the environment, or how often you've been exposed to a potentially addictive substance, can shift brain neurochemistry, increasing the likelihood of addiction.[20,21,26] Just as animals that are repeatedly given cocaine show a decrease in dopamine function, animals who are given high concentrations of sugar solutions also show changes in brain circuitry that promote addiction.[12] Likewise, when animal models are fed a cafeteria diet (a wide variety of highly palatable foods), their dopaminergic neurotransmission becomes depressed.[20] But they can *temporarily* restore dopamine levels if they eat

> If exposing ourselves to highly palatable foods can shift brain chemistry, then we clearly live in an environment perfectly designed to foster food addiction.

more of these foods. Thus, it becomes a vicious cycle. Current evidence indicates that compulsive behaviors, such as overeating, may be due to an interaction between nature (genetic susceptibility) and nurture (environment). So, if exposing ourselves to highly palatable foods can shift brain chemistry, then we clearly live in an environment perfectly designed to foster food addiction.

Controversy over the use of the term food addiction. The term "food addiction" is somewhat controversial. Some would ask, "How can a label of 'addictive' be applied to food, something which supports life itself?" Eating is necessary for survival; drugs of abuse obviously are not. However, while humans *do* need food to survive, what they do not need are excessive amounts of highly-palatable foods, which are so pervasive in our diets. And while the science linking food and drug addiction is still relatively young, the data that is emerging clearly supports the existence of an overlap between these behaviors.[30] Of course the food industry is not too keen on the term food addiction—the dreaded "A-word." For them,

> "Getting unhooked on foods is harder than getting unhooked on narcotics because you can't go cold turkey. You can't just stop eating."

the term addiction probably brings to mind images of strung-out junkies who hold up convenience stores at gunpoint for the money they need for another fix. Addiction also raises legal issues the industry would prefer to avoid. Thus, the food industry tries to defend itself by arguing that *true* narcotic addiction, for example, has specific technical thresholds that you just don't find in food addiction.[1] While, yes, what they're saying may be true, the reality is that today's processed foods are so cheap and readily available, there's simply no need to rob a store to get that "fix."

We often see the food industry point a finger at the consumer, blaming them for having a lack of self-control, instead of the industry accepting responsibility for deliberately making processed food addictive. But according to Dr. Nora Volkow, the Director of the National Institute on Drug Abuse (NIDA) at the National Institutes of Health, it's more difficult for people to control their eating habits than it is to control use of narcotics. Dr. Volkow explains, "Getting unhooked on foods may be harder than getting unhooked on narcotics, because you can't go cold turkey. You can't just stop eating."

While the food industry may claim they are simply trying to stay competitive by tweaking their products to entice us into buying, one could argue that that's simply no excuse for endangering the health of the public by developing new foods and drinks loaded with more sugar, salt, and fat to entice us to buy and eat more. In fact, during his interviews with scientists and executives of the big food companies, Michael Moss[1] discovered something quite interesting. By and large, these individuals admitted that they don't eat their own products (such as Cheetos® and Lunchables), nor do they serve them to their families. When Moss interviewed Howard Moskowitz, the man who reinvented Dr. Pepper,

> Scientists and executives of big food companies admit that they don't eat their own products. Why? They know better. They know about the addictive properties of sugar, salt, and fat.[1]

his signature drink, Moskowitz admitted: "I'm not a soda drinker. It's not good for your teeth." Clearly, the Food Giant scientists and executives know better. They know that consuming their products can cause severe health problems over the long run. They know about the addictive properties of sugar, salt, and fat, yet they work hard to make their products as irresistible as possible.

Chapter 2

What Makes Foods So Darn Tasty
(What Gives Certain Foods the Power to Hook Us)?

Generally speaking, we think of a food as being *palatable* if it tastes good. But when scientists say a food is palatable, they are referring to its capacity to prompt us and drive us, to eat more. So what exactly makes a food palatable?

1. **A high concentration of potent ingredients.** It appears that humans are hardwired, or have a built-in craving for sweet, fatty, and salty foods.[31] A preference for these substances was important for early humans because it encouraged them to seek out and consume safe and nutritious foods, such as ripe fruit. However, today, food manufacturers exploit this phenomenon by deliberately making

their products *extra*-sweet, fatty, or salty. The result? They amp up our neurons. The message to eat becomes stronger. We are driven to compulsively eat more and more of these potent foods. According to a review on sweeteners by Matte and Popkins:[32]

> Repeated exposure to a taste or flavor leads to increased acceptance for foods or beverages characterized by that taste or flavor. The desired intensity of the sensation is directly related to the concentration of the compounds responsible for the sensation.

Potent foods are typically those that have been *refined* by an industrial process. For example, the refining of carbohydrates allows for rapid digestion and, therefore, very rapid absorption. As a result, you have a surge of potentially psychoactive substances literally being dumped into the blood stream, which can, ultimately, alter our brain chemistry and get us hooked *(see **Figure 4**),*[22] a phenomenon similar to that seen with drug use. For example, coca leaves have been used since ancient times for their stimulating effects,

Figure 4. Both drugs and refined foods unnaturally stimulate our natural reward system

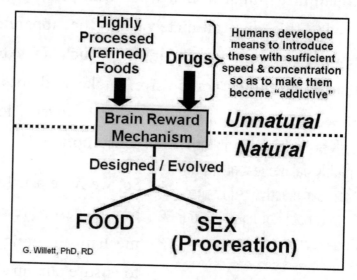

but people learned to purify or alter the leaves, producing cocaine that can be delivered more quickly to the brain by, for example, injecting or smoking it. This makes the drug more addictive. Food has evolved in a similar manner. Today, we refine and process our food so that, whereas our ancestors ate *whole* grains, today we're eating *refined* breads and cereals. While early Native Americans ate corn, we now consume corn syrup (or high-fructose corn syrup). The problem is that the consumption of potent processed or refined foods triggers an *excessive* release of dopamine, similar to that when using recreational drugs. This may ultimately alter the dopamine-reward function in the brain to such an extent that it promotes compulsive intake and loss of control over food consumption.[11,12]

> What's the link between drugs and highly palatable foods? Both act as psychoactive substances that are capable of hijacking our natural reward circuitry.

So, we have a natural brain pleasure-reward mechanism designed to ensure our survival and procreation (see **Figure 4**). But, because humans are so good at solving problems, we've figured out how to cheat the system—to trigger it to give us lots of dopamine quickly by using drugs. And we've taken whole foods—natural foods—and modified them (refined/processed/concentrated them) to a point where they *unnaturally* stimulate our natural reward system. Because these foods stimulate the very same part of our brain that responds to heroin and cocaine, it makes them very difficult to resist.

So, what's the link between drugs and highly palatable foods? Both act as psychoactive substances that are capable of high-jacking our natural reward circuitry. They tap into the very core systems that evolved to ensure survival. They arouse reward mechanisms artificially, in ways that were never meant to be. They are essentially "stolen pleasures" that may, ultimately, be disrupting the normal drive that was designed or evolved to protect us.

2. **Combining ingredients.** While most palatable foods contain sugar, fat, and salt, the art of pleasing the palate depends, in large part, on *combining* these ingredients in optimal amounts. According to David Kessler's book, *The End of Overeating*,[3] food is now being engineered to reach what the food industry refers to as the "bliss point" *(see Figure 5)*, which is the specific combination of sugar, fat, and salt that makes a product "hyperpalatable," precisely calculated to send the consumer over the moon! You can think of sugar, salt, and fat as three points of a compass

Figure 5. The Bliss Point

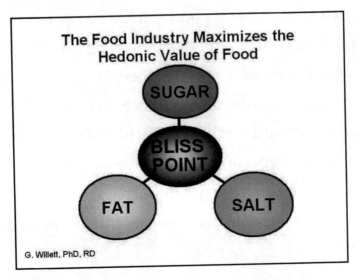

which, when perfectly combined, can make food overpoweringly compelling.

There is an enormous amount of scientific research and exquisite calibration that goes into tweaking the ratios of sugar, salt, and fat to achieve maximum bliss in a particular product. For example, as more sugar is added, the product becomes more pleasurable until the bliss point is reached. If it becomes too sweet, the level of pleasure drops off. But if a product succeeds in reaching the bliss point if it achieves just the right mix; the food becomes more stimulating and, to some people, irresistible. The bliss formula is one way that the processed food industry can effectively hook consumers. Multiple taste receptors, postingestive signals, and neuropeptide systems are activated,[26] stimulating our pleasure circuits so the drive to eat becomes stronger.

The bliss point is a powerful phenomenon. It dictates what we eat and drink more than we realize. Because when a food reaches the bliss point, it becomes more compelling. It becomes indulgent. It makes our Twinkie circuit light up. And because of that, consumption of this food may actually *stimulate* our appetite rather than *suppress* it. So, essentially, what the food industry is doing is combining substances in ways that are entirely *unnatural,* but which enhance their hedonic value, their addictive force.[3] One example of a food that combines ingredients to hit the bliss point is doughnuts, which contain refined flour, sugar, salt, and fat. Another is french fries, which contain carbs from potatoes, coupled with fat, salt, and often, dextrose. But the "king" of addictive foods is the potato chip.

> The bliss formula is one way that the processed food industry can effectively hook consumers.

"Bet you *can't* eat just one," one famous chip maker famously claimed. Potato chips contain the "holy trinity" of sugar, salt, and fat.[1] After being cut into thin slices, the potatoes are fried to a crisp, then generously bathed in salt. The moment you put one in your mouth, your tongue gets an instant hit from the salt that provides a burst of flavor. The potato starches are quickly converted to an easily digestible carbohydrate, or sugar, which enters your blood stream, causing your blood sugar to spike, and pleasure to be achieved. So what you have are combinations, in concentrations much larger than those found in nature, but that are dissociated from foods with nutritional value.[22] These combinations stimulate the drive to eat *more*.

3. **Variety.** Early humans lived as hunter-gatherers. They needed to obtain as much food as possible,

whenever it became available. One survival strategy was to select a wide variety of foods rather than depend on a few foods or a single food source. This provided an additional benefit because the more varied the human diet, the greater the likelihood of obtaining the wide variety of nutrients our bodies need for optimal functioning. As a consequence of these ancient survival strategies, people still respond to variety today by consuming greater total quantities of food when food is varied.[31]

Variety, or having a multisensory experience, amplifies eating.[33] We've known this to be the case since all the way back in the 1960s, when Anthony Sclafani, a then grad student at the University of Chicago, just by chance, put a rat on a lab bench near some fallen Froot Loops® (a multi-colored, multi-flavored, sugary cereal—in case you didn't know). Sclafani was struck by how fast the animal picked up the cereal and started to eat it. The rat was probably thinking: "How exciting, much better than that old chow they give me every day."

Well, Sclafani turned that casual observation into a formal experiment[34] giving rats what he called the "supermarket diet"—a wide *variety* of foods such as cookies, salami, cheese, bananas, marshmallows, peanut butter, and chocolate. Let's face it: Rats like a lot of the same foods we like. And what he found was that, after just 10 days, the animals fed the supermarket diet weighed significantly more than those fed the bland chow. And they continued to gain weight, becoming twice as heavy as their control counterparts. Sclafani concluded that feeding rats a variety of highly palatable supermarket foods was a particularly effective way of producing dietary obesity.[34] So we might ask, "Why did they keep eating? What happened to their homeostatic controls? How come they couldn't defend themselves against weight gain?"

When we have easy access to a *variety* of foods high in sugar, salt, and fat, our homeostatic biological system may go awry.[3] Clearly, the food industry is very aware of how attracted we are to variety. That's why it introduces thousands and thousands of new processed food products every year. Grocery stores exploit this phenomenon by devoting large amounts of shelf space to a wide variety of highly profitable, sugar-sweetened beverages, salty snacks, and dessert items. And, while the content may not vary that much from a nutritional standpoint, from the consumer's perspective there is tremendous variation in terms of packaging, labeling, flavors, colors, names, and other characteristics. And we may subconsciously interpret this as representing *nutritional* variety,[31] and thus have the drive to eat more.

There is a related concept called *sensory specific satiety*.[35] This is the tendency to stop eating and feel full or satisfied when variety is limited, but to do just the opposite, keep eating, when food is varied. When there is an abundance of different flavors at one meal or snack, the brain's appetite center tends to be overstimulated, so that we end up overeating,

> **Sensory Specific Satiety:**
> The tendency to stop eating and feel full when variety is limited, but continue to eat when food is varied.

well before our brain has a chance to tell us that we're full. It's not just a theory. It has been proven, at least in the hypothalamic neurons of monkeys.[36] If a monkey is presented with a food they've already had a lot of exposure to, their hypothalamic hunger neurons don't respond.[36] But when they are exposed to other, more novel foods, those neurons continue to respond. They continue to fire. And the animal wants more. Variety is not simply limited to flavor or taste (sweet, salty, sour, bitter). It can also pertain to color. Dr. Brian Wansink, author of the book *Mindless Eating*,[37] has shown that if people are offered 10 different colors of jellybeans, they'll eat about 43 percent more candies than if they are only offered a seven-color combination.[38] This is the case, even though they all taste pretty much the same. Even a variety in the shape of food plays a role. For example, people will eat more pasta if it is served in different shapes. And they'll eat the most pasta if it is served in different colors *and* shapes.[39]

So what is the take-home message? Will compulsive overeating go away if we just stick to gruel? One approach is to offer *less variety* of the things we want people to eat less of, such as sweets and salty snacks. But the flip-side is to offer *more variety* of things we want people to eat more of, such as fruits and vegetables. If a range of different colored fruits and vegetables are offered in a variety of different shapes, people are likely to eat more of them and benefit from the fiber, antioxidants, and phytochemicals they contain.

4. **Advertising and marketing.** While products may be knowingly engineered to maximize their allure, the advertising and marketing of the product plays a huge role. We know that environmental cues are very effective triggers for food cravings. Marketers use "priming" (e.g., images, sounds, smells, and even lighting) to prime people to be hungry or to desire their products, even when there is no physiological need for food.[31,40] The sight of food *alone* stimulates the secretion of dopamine in the mesolimbic system, which results in cravings and incentives to eat.[31] This neurophysiological response appears to be identical to what drug

addicts experience when shown images of their drugs of choice, although the response to food is clearly weaker. So, in other words, our external environment can trigger dopamine secretion and there's not much we can do about it. In today's modern society, we are essentially being *artificially* induced to feel hungry. And even if we don't see the food directly, we become conditioned by symbols or advertising logos. Research shows that such cues can modulate food-seeking behavior and food intake via classical conditioning.[19] We become conditioned just like the classic case of Pavlov and his dogs. Pavlov showed that when dogs were exposed to repeated pairing of a tone (sound) with a piece of meat, eventually the tone itself would elicit salivation in these animals.[19]

Brain imaging studies are now providing strong evidence that manufactured (processed) foods high in sugar, salt, and fat can "highjack" the brain in a way similar to drugs of abuse.

In a study using functional MRI in adolescents, it was shown that exposure to Coke® advertising activated gustatory and visual brain regions, with a greater response observed in those who were habitual Coke® consumers.[41] This finding suggests that the logo *itself* has become a conditioned cue. The authors concluded that habitual soft drink intake promotes hyper-responsivity of regions encoding salience/attention toward brand specific cues. This conditioned response then affects the motivation to consume the particular product. For example, maybe you had KFC™ chicken sometime in the past and experienced a pleasant dopamine reward. So your brain links the pleasure of that experience to, for example, the image of Colonel Sander's beard or that well-known red and white bucket. The more we experience the dopamine reward, the more salient (or prominent) that cue becomes. We eventually get to a point where all we have to do is see the logo and we find ourselves on autopilot. We want that food or drink! Clearly, the food industry is a master manipulator of consumers' minds and desires.

Today, food marketing and packaging is scientifically tailored to excite every one of our senses, using every psychological trick in the book. The advertising and food industry rely more and more on expertise from neuroscientists and psychologists. And the term "neuromarketing" is the new buzzword.[42] Who is their primary target? Kids. Neuromarketing to children is particularly profitable. Why? Because decisions made early on, especially in the teen years, will influence the development of brand loyalty. So, for example, a child that chooses Coke® or Pepsi® at age 13 or 14 is likely to maintain that brand loyalty throughout the rest of their lives. Michael Moss writes:

> Apart from the sugar, salt, and fat in their products, advertising is often the most powerful tool the industry has to create allure. Oftentimes it is the only thing companies can use to distinguish themselves from their competitors.[1]

You can clearly see the power of advertising in the cereal aisle today. High profit margins for cereal have led to severe overcrowding. There may be 200-plus cereal brands competing for your attention. For this reason, food manufacturers now spend nearly twice as much money on advertising their cereals than they do on the ingredients that go into them. A report from the

> The advertisement and food industry rely more and more on expertise from neuroscientists and psychologists. "Neuromarketing" is the new buzzword.

Federal Trade Commission exposed some of the industry's documents, such as an exuberant house ad in a magazine called *Broadcast* that offered some blunt advice for advertisers:

> If you're selling, Charlie's Mom is buying. But you've got to sell Charlie first. While his allowance is only 50 cents a week, his buying power is an American phenomenon. When Charlie sees something he likes, he usually gets it. Just ask General Mills or McDonald's. Of course, if you want Charlie, you have to catch him while he's sitting down. Or standing still. And that's not easy. Lucky for you, Charlie's into TV. And, of course, Charlie won't be watching alone! You'll also be reaching Jeff and Timmy, Chris and Susie, Mary, and his little brother John. That's what we mean by Kid Power.[1]

This knowledge should make us mad! The industry has a lot at stake when it comes to attracting our kids as their target customers. That's why they

> The food industry is the manipulator of consumers' minds and desires.

work so hard! In his book, Moss reveals just how ruthless food company executives and scientists are, not only in aggressively marketing junk food to children, but also to the poor. He fills his book with a plethora of damning examples. For example, his research uncovered how Coke® regularly preys on the poor and refers to its most loyal customers—in places like New Orleans and Rome, Georgia—as their "heavy users."[1] In Brazil, the company has been known to win over new customers in impoverished favelas (shanty towns) by repackaging its sugary beverage into smaller, 20-cent servings. Class division is clearly very apparent in the world of junk food marketing.

Chapter 3

What Foods Are Implicated in the Development of Food Addiction?

O f course, not *all* foods are addictive, but it is clear that *certain* foods have addictive qualities, and that eating these foods only makes us want to eat more and more of them. In general, addictive foods are those that raise dopamine levels the highest or the fastest. It's helpful to use a comparison with drugs because some drug rewards are more seductive than others. For example, methadone is less seductive and addictive than morphine, which is less seductive and addictive than heroin. Why? The relative addictive potency of a drug will differ based on the speed of action and rate of clearance. Methadone enters and leaves the brain more slowly than morphine, which, in turn, enters and leaves the brain more slowly than heroin. Presumably for this reason, methadone doesn't produce either the rapid high or the rapid withdrawal distress that we see with morphine and heroin. Likewise, the foods that have the greater tendency to be addictive (or seductive) are those that cause the most potent release/surge of dopamine. These are the ones that are most effective at targeting the pleasure center and giving you that "Aah" effect. And, even though they probably won't make you dance on a table or rob a convenience store, they might affect your brain just enough to get you hooked.

CHARACTERISTICS THAT RAISE THE ADDICTIVE POTENTIAL OF A FOOD

1. **Refined.** For most of human history, we survived on unadorned animal and vegetable products—meat, poultry, fish, beans, whole grains, vegetables, and fruit. We now subsist on foods that bear little resemblance to what exists in nature. Let's face it—edible food-like substances are no longer products of nature, but products of food science. I tell people if your Grandma

> Edible food-like substances are no longer products of nature, but products of food science.

wouldn't recognize it, don't eat it! What we're talking about here are foods that are *refined* by an industrial process, such as sugar and other sweeteners, flour, salt, and certain fats. Like drugs, these ingredients do not become addictive until they are extracted and concentrated by modern industrial processes. For example, the refining of carbohydrates allows for rapid digestion and, therefore, very rapid absorption. So we have a surge of potentially psychoactive substances dumped into the blood stream, which can ultimately alter our brain chemistry and even change our moods. So we demand more and more. We become like the heroin addict. We can't go without it. Instead, we want unrefined carbohydrates that are digested and absorbed slowly. So that, just like methadone, they go through the system more slowly, and therefore produce less compulsive intake.

> An easy rule of thumb is that if your grandma wouldn't recognize the food, you probably shouldn't be eating it!

2. **Potent.** Foods that have a high concentration of rewarding ingredients,

such as sugar *(see **Chapter 5**, page 65)*, give us a blast of dopamine, causing our Twinkie circuitry to just light up. In fact, animal studies have shown that sweet foods have a higher reinforcing value than cocaine, even in animals with an extensive history of drug intake.[43] Now, clearly, sugar is found in natural, healthy foods, but the difference is that, in healthier foods, sugar (1) is found in smaller concentrations, and (2) coexists with other substances found in natural foods, such as fiber, vitamins, and trace minerals that serve the useful purpose. But today, manufacturers often add lots and lots of sugar to hit that "sweet spot"— to make us crave more and more of that food. The industry also puts tons of fat *(see **Chapter 7**, page 129)* in foods because fat is responsible for the characteristic texture, flavor, and aroma of many foods, and largely determines the palatability of the diet. It also promotes the release of flavor-enhancing chemicals. Fat helps flavor merge and meld, creating a smooth sensation.

3. **Ingredients combined in unnatural ways that enhance their addictive forces.** As described earlier, prime examples of these artificial combinations include doughnuts and French fries. In his book,[3] Dr. Kessler describes research in which animals would get a sugar reward for pressing a lever once. Next, six lever pushes were needed to get a second reward, then 10, 16, and 23 pushes to get the third, fourth, and fifth rewards. The researchers were looking for that breaking point—the point at which the animals would just give up, figuring it wasn't worth it anymore. They found that animals will generally work harder, or press the lever more times, in order to get more rewards. But they will also work harder to get higher concentrations of a sugar reward. For example, in order to get a highly-prized reward of a 20 percent sugar solution, rats would press the lever as many as 44 times! But there was a limit to their desire for sweetness. They actually worked less hard when the sugar concentrations exceeded 30 percent sugar. We see the same phenomenon with fat. When Dr. Sara Ward was at the University of North Carolina at

> Animals will work for a combined sugar-fat reward almost as hard as they will for a cocaine reward.

Chapel Hill, she would have her animals poke their noses into holes a certain number of times to get a fat reward (a corn oil solution). She found that a 10 percent corn oil solution had the greatest reinforcing properties. Animals would poke their noses into a hole 50 times to earn that reward. But, her work clearly showed that animals will work the hardest for a reward consisting of a *combination* of fat and sugar. In fact, animals will work for a combined sugar-fat reward almost as hard as they will for a cocaine reward.[4] And if you add in salt *(see **Chapter 9**, page 215)*, the bliss point is achieved as the food becomes more stimulating. We're a lot like those rats. When we are given that unnatural combination, our brains are stimulated (super-charged), and we want more and more and more.

Thus, in general, "addictive" foods are those that are highly potent and highly palatable combinations of fats, sugars, and salt. Moreover, these foods are generally comprised of synthetic (refined) combinations of ingredients that may make them potentially more addictive than traditional foods.[44] You can think of addictive foods as foods that were "made in a plant rather than grown on a plant." It's harder to imagine someone binging on a whole bowl of apples or corn than someone gorging on a whole bag of chips or cookies.

Fast food appears to have many attributes that increase their salience, or their "pull." The majority of fast food meals are accompanied by a soda, which increases the sugar content 10-fold. The high fat and salt content of fast food also increase its addictive potential. Finally, fast food advertisements, restaurants, and menus all provide highly enticing environmental cues that may trigger addictive overeating. While the concept of fast food addiction remains to be proven, more and more research supports the role of fast food as a potentially addictive substance that is most likely to create dependence, particularly in vulnerable populations.[45]

So, why can't we just say "no" to addictive foods? Well, first of all, addictive foods are everywhere, they're convenient, and they're marketed with such compelling advertising. It's hard to resist. A second part of the reason is denial. A lot of people don't know much about nutrition. And other people don't really *want* to know more about nutrition, in part because they're resistant to changing eating patterns. "Don't you tell me what to eat!" Sometimes I think the general population just doesn't really want to hear about how destructive these foods are to our health and well-being. How many people watched Morgan Spurlock's health decline in the documentary film, *Super Size Me*, and were briefly spooked, but then went on to continue with their fast food ways? A third reason that we just can't say "no" is that we have become overpowered by the food industry. According to Dr. Kessler's book, *The End of Overeating*,[3] the industry has "cracked the code of conditioned hypereating." They know exactly how to manipulate our eating behavior, so they can sell more and more of their products.

> Generally speaking, addictive foods are foods that were made in a plant rather than grown on a plant.

Chapter 4

Combatting **Nutritionism**:
The Whole Foods Approach

Food is a primal, everyday part of our lives— yet rich with mystery. It seems there are more questions than answers. But today, nutritional science is on the cusp of a revolution. Since the late nineteenth century, nutrition science has been characterized by the attempt to understand food and diets in terms of their nutrient and biochemical composition. Thus, the gold standard of nutrition research has been to break down food into its individual, constituent parts, or nutrients. This reductionist paradigm is referred to as *nutritionism*,[46] an ideology that has dominated nutritional science, dietary advice, and food marketing for decades. However, the problem with this nutrient-by-nutrient approach is that it takes the nutrient out of the context of food, the food out of the context of diet, and the diet out of the context of lifestyle.[47] When, in reality, food, diet, and culture are extremely complicated processes that can't possibly be isolated into single variables to be studied.

When we focus on *individual* nutrients as the key indicators of what makes a food healthy, we may end up ignoring subtle interactions *between* nutrients. We may overlook the fact that the *whole* may be more than, or maybe just *different* from, the sum of its parts. Take an apple for example. Every apple contains thousands of antioxidants, with names that might seem quite foreign to us. But each of these powerful chemicals has the potential to play an important role in supporting our health by impacting thousands upon thousands of metabolic reactions inside the human body. If we attempt to isolate and calculate the specific influence of each of these chemicals, it just simply isn't going to be possible to determine the effect of the apple as a *whole*. And since almost *every* chemical can affect every *other* chemical, there are an almost infinite number of possible biological consequences. This may explain why, for example, fruits and vegetables, *as a whole*, have been shown to decrease the risk of cancer in epidemiological studies, but studies on an *isolated* nutrient, such as beta-carotene (a carotenoid found in fruits and vegetables), have, paradoxically, found it to be harmful, rather than helpful, in relationship to cancer. That's because beta-carotene, *isolated*, is not the same as beta-carotene in the context of the whole carrot. The carrot is helpful; the isolated beta-carotene is not. In his new book, *Whole*,[48] Dr. T. Collin Campbell explains how *nutritionism* is problematic because it ignores the fascinating complexity of the human body and provides little insight into the complexity of what really happens in our bodies, or how those nutrients/chemicals contribute to our health.

Perhaps even more problematic, this narrow, reductionist approach has often distorted our appreciation of food quality and, in some cases, even benefited food manufacturers by allowing them to promote their foods, even highly processed foods, as "healthy" on the basis of their quantity of "good" or "bad" nutrients. Thus, nutritionism has become a powerful means by which the food industry can strategically promote their nutritionally/chemically enhanced "edible food-like substances" as "good for us," using a wide range of health claims as marketing tools. Nutritionism has essentially adapted our minds and bodies to the nutritional marketing strategies and nutritionally engineered products of the food industry. It has aligned the demands and perceived needs of consumers with the commercial interests of food manufacturers.[49]

Let's face it. The average consumer really doesn't understand the concepts of saturated fat and dietary fiber. They might look at the packaging and see words like "high fiber" and "good source of vitamin C," and thus assume that the product is "healthy, "even though the fiber or vitamin could have simply been *added* to the product. The reality may be that it is, for the most part, a highly-processed, synthetic food.

So, while the advice to consume a largely plant-based diet (fruits, vegetables, and grains) has not really changed much over the past 50 years, the fact of the matter is that people have become increasingly confused about what they are supposed to eat to stay healthy. In her book, *Food Politics: How the Food Industry Influences Nutrition and Health,*[47] Marion Nestle examined how, over the years, the food industry lobbied the U.S. government to shape official dietary guidelines in ways that undermined criticism of processed foods, and of high meat and dairy consumption. For example, dietary guidelines recommend that we eat less of particular *nutrients*, such as saturated fat and sugar, rather than less of the *actual foods* that contain high levels of these nutrients, such as fatty meat or processed sweets. And, along the way, as food has been replaced by nutrients, it seems as though common sense has been replaced by confusion. According to a recent food and health survey, 52 percent of Americans polled believe it's easier to do their taxes than to figure out how to eat healthfully.[47] Nestle argues that the food industry has created a state of *nutrition confusion*, which is distorting the view of what food *should* be. It is shaping our relationship to food and to our bodies, and heightening our nutritional anxieties in the process. By promoting poor quality, hyperpalatable foods on one hand, and creating an environment that confuses the basic principles of diet and health on the other, the food industry is, ultimately, contributing to overeating and poor nutritional practices.

One might also argue that the scientific process and, especially, the way that research studies are represented (or often misrepresented) to the public, by way of the media, is also adding to the state of nutrition confusion. We hear that a low-fat diet helps with weight loss, but that a high-carb diet makes us fat. So what can we eat? The next week we may hear similar advice, except that it is completely flipped around to instead recommend a high-fat, low-carb diet…or maybe we just can't remember. It's so confusing! One week we hear about a study extolling the benefits of fish oil, but the next week, the nightly news starts off with a report claiming that it causes cancer. Butter one week, margarine the next. Milk, no milk. Eggs, no eggs. One year we hear about strict guidelines to lower sodium, then we hear a major health organization saying that maybe all those restrictions were not necessary after all. And we think,

"Can't anyone make up their minds? HELP!!" We hear things like paleo-diet, detox diet, blood-type diet, alkaline diet, and vegan diet. Don't eat anything that had a face or came from something that had a face. What??? Can anyone simplify this barrage of often conflicting information?

Unfortunately, most people don't understand that science, especially nutritional science, is a slow process of testing hypotheses, retesting, throwing out ideas, adding new ones, etc. What we are looking for is a *body* of scientific evidence that supports a given hypothesis. No one study, by itself, is sufficient. We have to look at the *totality* of the evidence. Moreover, different study designs, whether observational epidemiological studies or randomized control trials, whether human or animal, they all have their strengths and weakness. But the uninformed public, wanting a quick and easy answer, simply doesn't understand the process. They get frustrated with the seemingly contradictory information. Plus, you have opposing sides and political forces (e.g., meat and dairy industries and large multi-national food companies) getting their hands into the pot, lobbying to make their voices/their perspectives heard, trying to persuade us with their political clout and expensive advertising schemes. But, in the end, we're the ones who suffer. We're the losers. We're the ones feeling confused, with our hands up in the air thinking, "If you top experts can't agree, then I guess it doesn't matter what I eat! Let them eat cake! Why can't we just get along?"

So what is the solution? Instead of thinking of foods in terms of particular nutrients, perhaps a better course of action would be to focus on consuming more *whole foods* to replace the processed, refined, fake foods that capitalize the marketplace. In an ideal world, we would all be eating whole foods that don't rely on plastic packaging and a long list of mysterious ingredients that sound more like something concocted in a chemistry lab, rather than actual food. Michael Pollan recommends that we focus on *real* foods, ones with ingredients that are recognizable and that don't rely on health claims.[2] This will enable us to break free from the Food Giants and change the way we view food and nutrition, and take steps to reclaim our health.

So, forgive me, in advance, for providing detailed information, for example, on specific types of dietary sugars and fatty acids, in the remainder of this book. My intent is to expose the many contradictions and controversies in the field of nutrition—no matter how frustrating they tend to be. But, while I provide this as background information, my overarching goal in writing this book is to encourage you to change your overall approach to food: to limit the processed, addictive, edible *food-like* substances that are the products of food science, and instead to consume *whole, real foods* that are products of nature. This is an approach that is not only good for your body and mind, but good for the planet as well.

Chapter 5

Sugar

The first thing to know about sugar is this: it has a primal pull. Our bodies are hard-wired to crave sweet foods. Infants who are given drops of sugar water exhibit pleasurable facial expressions. And the sweeter the solution, the more they like it. Even bacteria swim toward sugar. It's a very ancient motivation. And we now know that our ability to detect sugar or sweet taste is a lot more complicated than we once thought.

Taste occurs when specific proteins in the food bind to receptors on taste buds. These receptors, in turn, send messages to the brain's cerebral cortex, which interprets the flavor. Do you remember that tongue diagram that supposedly maps out the specific locations where our main tastes (sweet, salty, bitter, sour) are detected? Well, it turns out that the tongue map was wrong! It is a mistranslation of an early-1900s German thesis that was disproved in 1974 (even though, unfortunately, it continues to be published in textbooks today). The fact of the matter is that we perceive *all* taste qualities *all over* our tongue. Each taste bud actually has receptors for sweet, sour, salty, and bitter sensations, though there may be increased sensitivity to certain qualities/tastes in certain areas.[50] Continued research into this intricate biological process has revealed a complex neural and chemical network such that our taste buds are sensitive to a complex flavor spectrum, similar to how our vision is sensitive to a broad color spectrum grouped into four major colors (red, orange, yellow, and green). However, when it comes to sugar/sweet taste, it appears that the entire mouth goes absolutely wild! When those sweet receptors in the mouth's 10,000 taste buds detect the sensation of sweetness, they send a message of pleasure directly to the brain. But the excitement doesn't stop there. We now know that the receptors that sense sugar (and even artificial sweeteners) can be found all the way down our esophagus, into the stomach and even in the pancreas. That means that our gut and pancreas can detect sweet foods and drinks with receptors that are virtually identical to those in the mouth. In fact, our appetite for sweet flavors is actually *enhanced* by the post-oral reinforcing actions of the sugars in the gut and beyond.[51] Such advancements have led to the development of a new field of study called *gastrointestinal chemosensation*, which is working to understand how cells of the gut detect and respond to sugars, as well as other nutrients, and the ways in which these cells/receptors are intricately linked to our appetites.[52]

Our innate preference for sweetness has protective value because, in nature, a sweet taste generally signaled a good source of safe calories (such as ripe fruit). And, contrary to popular opinion, our drive toward sweet flavors should not necessarily lead to obesity or other diet-related diseases. That's because sugar-containing foods in their *natural* form (e.g., in fruits) actually tend to be highly nutritious, and contain beneficial vitamins, minerals, and phytochemicals. Moreover, such foods elicit a high level of satiety (relative to calories they contain) because of their high-fiber content, low-energy density, and low glycemic load *(see section, "QUALITY carbs," page 103)*. It is only when sugars are refined, concentrated, and consumed in large amounts that they can become problematic.

Clearly, today, manufacturers are taking advantage of America's sweet tooth by adding as much sugar/sweeteners as possible. In fact, practically everything on American food shelves that can be sweetened, has been sweetened. In an attempt to increase sales, companies have been lacing once-wholesome foods such as yogurt and spaghetti sauce with astonishing amounts of sugar and sodium. For example, regular Yoplait yogurt contains twice as much sugar per serving as Lucky Charms, and half a cup of Prego Traditional spaghetti sauce has as much sugar as three Oreos. You might wonder, "Why do food manufacturers pack their products with so much sugar?" Well, not only does sugar make food tasty, sugar is also capable of pulling off a string of manufacturing miracles—from enhancing preservation, to conferring certain functional attributes, such as viscosity, texture, body, and browning capacity. For example, sugar makes donuts fry up bigger and gives cereal a toasty-brown color.[1] But at what price?

In the past, sugar was viewed quite favorably, with manufacturers eagerly touting it in their foods using a long list of euphemisms (such as: "honeyed", "sugarcoated," "sweet," "candied"). As a child, my favorite cereal, when I could get my hands on it, was Super Sugar Crisp. But the landscape changed drastically with the surge in obesity rates in the 1980s. In 1986, Professor J. Yudkin wrote a book devoted to sugar entitled, *Pure, White and Deadly*.[53] So what exactly is sugar, and is it really harmful if it is consumed in excess? Here are various definitions for sugars *(see **Table 1**)*. Some are based on the chemical structure of sugars *(**Table 2**)*. Our bodies can only absorb **mono**saccharides, or single sugars, which are the smallest sugar units. Most sugars found naturally

Table 1. Common definitions of sugars[54]

SIMPLE CARBOHYDRATES	Monosaccharides and disaccharides. Monosaccharides include *glucose, galactose,* and *fructose.* Dextrose is synonymous with glucose. *Fructose* is the most common naturally-occurring monosaccharide, and is found in fruits and vegetables. Common disaccharides include *sucrose* (glucose plus fructose), which is found in sugar cane, sugar beets, honey, and corn syrup; *lactose* (glucose plus galactose), found in milk products; and *maltose* (glucose plus glucose), found in malt.
COMPLEX CARBOHYDRATES	Glucose-containing polysaccharides, such as starch.
NATURALLY-OCCURRING (INTRINSIC) SUGARS	Sugars that are an integral part of whole fruit, vegetable, and milk products.
ADDED (EXTRINSIC) SUGARS	Sugars and syrups added to foods during processing or preparation; includes sugars and syrups added at the table.
TOTAL SUGARS	All sugars (naturally-occurring and added) in foods and beverages.
HIGH-FRUCTOSE CORN SYRUP	is produced from corn syrup, which undergoes enzymatic processing to increase the fructose content and is then mixed with glucose.

in foods or added to foods are **di**saccharides, or double sugars. For example, sucrose (table sugar) is glucose plus fructose. Lactose, found in dairy products, is glucose plus galactose. During digestion, these disaccharides are broken down by digestive enzymes into individual monosaccharides, which can

Table 2. Chemical structure of sugars

MONOSACCHARIDES *(single sugars)*	• Glucose • Fructose • Galactose
DISACCHARIDES *(double sugars)*	• Maltose = Glucose + Glucose • Sucrose = Glucose + Fructose • Lactose = Glucose + Galactose
POLYSACCHARIDES *(also known as starches or complex carbohydrates)*	• contain hundreds of single sugars

then be absorbed by the body. Starches or complex carbohydrates are polysaccharides, which contain hundreds of single sugars. It usually takes longer for the body to break down complex carbohydrates into monosaccharides for absorption.

Intrinsic vs. extrinsic sugars. Another way to classify sugars is based on whether they are *intrinsic* or *extrinsic*. Intrinsic sugars are defined as sugars that are present within the cell walls of plants (i.e., naturally-occurring), whereas extrinsic sugars are typically *added* to foods.

Added sugars. While sugars are naturally found in fruits and vegetables (in the form of fructose) and

Figure 6. *Sources of added sugar in U.S. Diet, for persons 2 years of age and older*

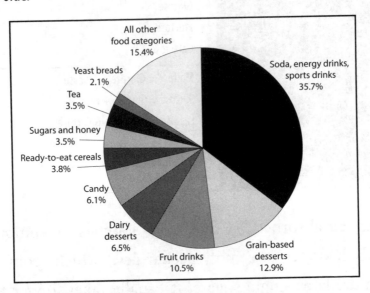

Source: 2010 USDA Dietary Guidelines for Americans.[55]

milk products (in the form of lactose), the majority of sugars found in the typical American diet are those that are *added* to foods. "Added sugars" are defined as sugars and syrups that are added to foods during processing or preparation, including sugars and syrups added at the table,[55] such as what you would find in soft drinks, candy, cakes, cookies, pies, cereals, and even pasta sauce. This does not refer to those sugars that are naturally occurring sugars, such as those in milk and whole fruit. Specifically, added sugars include white sugar, brown sugar, raw sugar, corn syrup, corn-syrup solids, high-fructose corn syrup, malt syrup, maple syrup, pancake syrup, fructose sweetener, liquid fructose, honey, molasses, anhydrous dextrose, and crystal dextrose.[55] *Figure 6* shows the sources of added sugar in the American diet, based on data from the National Health and Nutrition Examination Survey (NHANES) 2005–2006.[55] As can be seen in *Figure 6*, soft drinks and other sugar-sweetened beverages are, by far, the largest source of added sugars in Americans' diets, accounting for about 35.7 percent of our total added sugar intake. Although added sugars are not chemically different from naturally-occurring sugars, many foods and beverages that are major sources of added sugars have significantly lower micronutrient densities than foods and beverages that contain naturally-occurring sugars.

How much added sugar are we consuming? Table 3 lists the usual individual intake of added sugar by age. According to the National Health and Nutrition Examination Survey (NHANES) data (2001–2004),

Table 3. *Usual intake of added sugars (in teaspoonfuls), U.S. Population, 2001–2004*

	Age (in years)	Mean (tsp)
All persons	≥1	22.2
	1–3	12.2
	4–8	21.0
Males	9–13	29.2
	14–18	34.3
	≥1	25.4
Females	9–13	23.2
	14–18	25.2
	≥19	18.3

Source: National Cancer Institute. Usual intake of added sugars. In: Usual Dietary Intakes: Food Intakes, U.S. Population 2001–04. November 2008.[56]

the mean intake of added sugars for all persons aged one year or older is 22.2 teaspoons (about 355 calories) per day. However, 14- to 18-year-old males have the highest intake, at 34.3 teaspoons (about 549 calories) per day.[56] In general, U.S. children and adolescents consume an average of 16 percent of their daily calorie intake from added sugars.[57] One problem is that, currently, U.S. food labels list information on "total" sugars per serving, but do not distinguish between sugars that are naturally present in foods and those that are added. Thus, it is difficult for consumers to determine the amount of added sugars they are actually consuming.

High glycemic load carbohydrates. Glycemic load is a variable that assesses how a carbohydrate-containing food influences blood glucose levels. A glycemic load of more than 20 is considered to be "high;" a glycemic load of less than 10 is considered to be "low." In general, refined or processed carbohydrates tend to be high in glycemic load. For tables of the glycemic loads of common foods, see: *www.mendosa.com/gilists.htm.* Over the past few decades, there has been a global shift toward increased consumption of high glycemic load or refined carbohydrates foods, with detrimental effects on health.

Problems Associated with Excess Intake of Added Sugars/High Glycemic Load Foods

Impact on children's taste preferences. Kids love sugar and, often times, the sweeter, the better. However, basic research on taste in children is revealing evidence that by promoting extra sweet foods, the food industry is essentially shaping taste preferences in our kids. They are, in effect, teaching our children how sweet food *should* be. In doing so, it has been argued that the food industry is manipulating or

> By promoting extra sweet foods, the food industry is essentially shaping taste preferences in our kids. They are, in effect, teaching our children how sweet food should be.

exploiting the biology of children.[1] And, because of this, they are potentially impacting the long-term health of our children.

Excess energy intake/ weight gain. Over the past few decades, obesity has emerged as a major global health problem. In the United States, the percentage of overweight and obese adults increased markedly from 47 percent and 15 percent, respectively, from 1976 through 1980, to more than 66 percent and 33 percent from 2005 through 2006.[58] Over the same time period, total calorie intake in the United States has increased by an average of 150 to 300 calories per day, with approximately 50 percent of this increase coming from sugar-sweetened beverages, the primary source of added sugars in our diets.[54,59,60]

America's obesity epidemic has made it apparent that we need to match energy intake with energy expenditure. To accomplish this, it is important to monitor the amount of *discretionary* calories

Figure 7. *Comparison of the calories from nutrient-dense form of foods vs. additional calories from added sugars or solid fats*

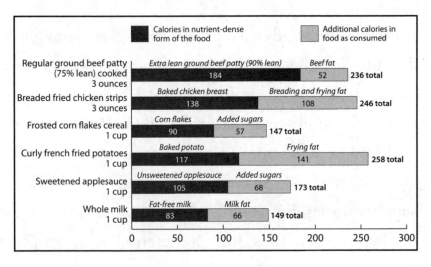

Source: USDA 2010 Dietary Guidelines for Americans.[55]

we consume. Total caloric intake is the sum of *essential* calories (the total energy intake needed to meet recommended nutrient intakes) and discretionary calories (the *additional* calories necessary to meet energy demands and for normal growth). Discretionary calories consist of solid fats (those with a high percentage of saturated and/or trans fatty acids that are solid at room temperature) and added sugars. ***Figure 7*** shows some examples of the calories in food choices that are not nutrient-dense and the calories in nutrient-dense forms of these foods.[55]

Although the body's response to sugars does not depend on whether they are *naturally* present or *added* to foods, sugars found naturally in foods are part of the food's total package of nutrients and other healthful components. In contrast, many processed and refined foods that contain added sugars often supply calories, but few or no essential nutrients and no dietary fiber. Thus, they are referred to as "empty calorie foods."

In the U.S. Department of Agriculture (USDA) old Food Guide Pyramid,[61] added sugars were placed at the tip of the pyramid, and consumers were advised to use them *sparingly* because they provide calories and little else. They can be included in your diet *only if* you have calories to spare after eating nutritious meals during the day, including plenty of fruits and vegetables, whole grains, low-fat dairy products, and lean proteins. According to the Dietary Guidelines for Americans,[55] most people should consume no more than 5 to 15 percent of calories from solid fats and added sugars. The American Heart Association[54] is more specific. They recommend that no more than **50 percent** of your discretionary calorie allowance should come from added sugar.

To meet these guidelines:

- a 1,200-calorie diet would be limited to no more than 16 grams (4 teaspoons) of added sugar per day

- a 1,800-calorie diet would be limited to no more than 20 grams (5 teaspoons) of added sugar per day

- a 2,400-calorie diet would be limited to no more than 48 grams (12 teaspoon) of added sugar per day

To simplify these recommendations, the American Heart Association[54] has set a *prudent upper limit* (maximum amount) of added sugar intake: most American women should eat or drink no more than 100 calories (about 6 teaspoons) per day, and most American men should eat or drink no more than 150 calories (about 9 teaspoons) per day of added sugars.[54] Well, if you consider that one 12-ounce can of soda contains at least 8 teaspoons of sugar, you'd have to limit yourself to one regular can of soda per day to meet this limit. That's clearly not a sweet deal for those fond of their colas or Mountain Dews. But, as you can see in *Table 3*, we're not doing so well by these guidelines. Current intakes far exceed the allowance for discretionary calories.

> The American Heart Association has set a prudent upper limit of intake for added sugars. They state that most American women should eat or drink no more than 100 calories per day (about 6 tsp) from added sugars, and most American men should eat or drink no more than 150 calories per day (about 9 tsp) from added sugars.[54]

Reducing the consumption of added sugars *(see Table 3)*, especially from sweetened beverages, has the advantage of lowering the calorie content of the diet, without compromising its nutrient adequacy.

Sugar-sweetened beverages (SSBs) and weight gain. During the past 30 years, there has been a marked increase in the consumption of SSBs (soft drinks, fruit drinks, and fruit punch) across the globe. As stated previously, about 50 percent of the increase in our caloric intake over the past three decades can be attributed to what we drink.[54] In the late 1970s, only 3.9 percent of total calories came from SSBs; by 2001, it had gone up to 9.2 percent, a three-fold increase).[62] Part of the blame rests on the supersizing of the beverage industry. While years past we mostly drank the 12-ounce can with its 9 teaspoons of sugar, as the obesity crisis was building in the 1980s, those cans gave way to 20-ounce bottles, with 15 teaspoons of sugar; and the 64-ounce Double Gulp sold by the 7-Eleven stores, with a whopping 44 teaspoons of sugar. Research in humans has linked SSBs to weight gain, particularly visceral obesity (the belly fat located beneath your abdominal muscles).[58] A prospective study involving middle-school students over the course of two academic years showed that the risk of becoming obese increased by 60 percent for every additional serving of sugar-sweetened beverages consumed per day.[63] In an 80-year prospective study involving women, those who increased their consumption of sugar-sweetened beverages at year four (and maintained this increase) gained 8 kg, whereas those who decreased their intake of sugar-sweetened beverages at year four (and maintained this decrease) gained only 2.8 kg.[64]

Why do SSBs promote weight gain? There may be several reasons.[58] First of all, sugar is highly palatable. Excessive consumption of sugar can trigger an exaggerated release of dopamine, which can promote a compulsive drive to consume *more* SSBs. This can lead to weight gain because SSBs contain a large amount of empty calories. Second, because they are liquid ("liquid candy"), they do not provide the same degree of satiety that solid calories do. There is evidence that our bodies simply do not recognize calories in liquids the same way they do calories in a solid form.[54,65] In fact, quite the opposite may occur. The rapidly absorbable carbohydrates in SSBs contribute to a high glycemic load, which is thought to actually stimulate appetite[58] *(see section, "High Glycemic Load," page 86)*. Finally, SSBs may also affect body weight through other behavioral mechanisms. For example, whereas the intake of solid food is characteristically coupled to hunger, people may consume SSBs in the absence of hunger, to satisfy thirst or for social reasons. SSBs may also have chronic adverse effects on taste preferences and food acceptance.[66] Persons (especially children) who

Figure 8. Effects of sugar-sweetened beverages on health

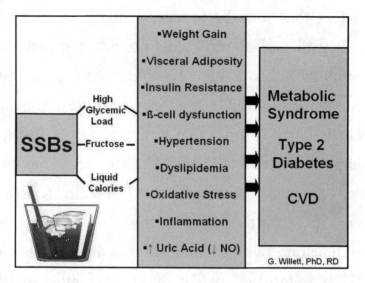

regularly consume sugar-sweetened beverages rather than water may find less sweet foods (e.g., fruits, vegetables, and legumes) unappealing or unpalatable. As a result, their diets may be of poor quality.

Excess sugar intake and chronic disease risk. Per capita consumption of refined foods has increased dramatically over the past several decades, and, in parallel, so has a range of metabolic abnormalities.[22] SSBs, the primary source of added sugars in the U.S. diet, are linked to other health consequences besides weight gain *(see Figure 8).*[54,58] Research shows that SSBs may increase the risk for metabolic syndrome, type 2 diabetes, and cardiovascular disease (CVD), an effect that may be independent of its effects on weight gain and obesity. SSBs provide high amounts of rapidly absorbable carbohydrates (i.e., high glycemic load), often in the form of fructose (or high-fructose corn syrup), that are typically consumed in large quantities. A high intake of SSBs has been linked to hyperinsulinemia and insulin resistance (even in children[67]); impaired ß-cell function, hypertension; dyslipidemia (high triglycerides, low HDL-cholesterol);[68] oxidative stress; inflammation; and increased uric acid levels (perhaps because the metabolism of fructose in the liver leads to the production of uric acid, which reduces the availability of nitric oxide).[69] Ultimately, these factors increase the risk for chronic disease. In a cross-sectional study[70] of U.S. adolescents enrolled in NHANES, high added sugar consumption was associated with high triglycerides and low HDL-cholesterol, as well as insulin resistance. The authors concluded that consumption of added sugars is positively associated with multiple measures that increase CVD risk. In the Framingham Offspring Study,[71] which followed 6,154 adults for four years, it was found that individuals who consumed one or more soft drinks per day had a 22 percent higher incidence of hypertension (135/85 mmHg or higher or being treated) compared with nonconsumers. Similarly, in the Nurses' Health Studies I and II,[72] women who consumed four or more SSBs per day had a 44 percent and 28 percent higher risk of incident hypertension, respectively, compared with infrequent consumers. The International Study of Macro/Micronutrients and Blood Pressure (INTERMAP)[73] showed that not only was SSB consumption associated with elevated blood pressure, but that, interestingly, this effect was stronger in people who consumed more sodium. This suggests that if you consume a high-sodium diet, you might be more sensitive to the possible blood pressure raising effects of SSBs. Regarding blood lipids, daily soft drink consumers in the Framingham Offspring Study[71] were found to have a 22 percent higher incidence of hypertriglyceridemia and low HDL-cholesterol compared with nonconsumers. In addition, high soft drink consumption has been associated with hyperuricemia[74] and risk of developing gout.[75]

> The 2011 American Heart Association guidelines for the prevention of cardiovascular disease in women recommend no more than 450 calories per week from sugar-sweetened beverages.[77]

It is clear that SSB consumption is linked to multiple risk factors for disease. Recently, in the Nurses' Health Study,[76] SSB intake was positively associated with the risk of coronary heart disease (CHD; nonfatal myocardial infarction or fatal CHD), even after accounting for the possible confounding effect of other unhealthy lifestyle factors. In the more than 88,000 women who were followed for 24 years in this study, those who consumed two or more SSBs per day had a 35 percent greater risk of developing CHD compared with those who consumed less than one SSB per month. The most recent guidelines put out by the American Heart Association for the prevention of cardiovascular disease in women recommend no more than 450 calories per week from SSBs.[77]

HIGH GLYCEMIC LOAD/REFINED CARBOHYDRATES & OVEREATING

Current evidence suggests that high glycemic load foods, or highly processed carbohydrates, such as white bread, potatoes, and concentrated sugars, can actually make us hungrier. They alter brain activity in ways that make us crave them even more. We know from animal research that rats that are given access to sweet cereal become so determined to get another portion that they will overcome their instinctual fear of open spaces, leave the safe confines of their cages, and travel out to an open field in order to get another chance to splurge on something sweet. In the extreme, rats that have been conditioned to expect an electrical shock when they eat cheesecake will still lunge for it. In fact, when access is unlimited, these animals will eat to a point of obesity.[77.1] It appears that their craving for sweets/refined carbohydrates completely overrides the biological brakes that *should* tell them to stop.

In a ground-breaking study,[78] researchers gave overweight or obese men test meals comprised of milkshakes that were either low or high glycemic load. After consuming the shakes, researchers measured the subjects' blood glucose levels and hunger, while, at the same time, using functional magnetic imaging (fMRI) to observe brain activity over a four-hour

> Refined carbohydrates may trigger overeating. The clear take-home message is that by limiting highly refined carbohydrates, we can help people avoid overeating.

period—a critical time period that influences eating behavior at the next meal. They found that, compared to the low glycemic load milkshake, the high glycemic load shake ultimately decreased blood sugar, made subjects hungrier, and triggered intense activation of the nucleus accumbens, the critical brain region involved in reward and cravings, and linked to substance abuse and dependence. This is the first time a study has so convincingly demonstrated that the biological effects of refined carbohydrates can provoke symptoms related to addiction, independent of calories and tastiness, in susceptible people (those who are overweight or obese). This may explain the strong link between the increased consumption of highly processed foods and soft drinks and rising obesity rates. The clear take-home message is that by avoiding highly processed/refined/high glycemic load carbohydrates, we can help people avoid overeating.

Is one type of sugar better (or worse) than another?
The bottom line is that sugar is sugar. Although brown sugar may be less processed than white sugar (or it may have had molasses added to change the color and flavor), the fact of the matter is that brown sugar is still sucrose, just like white sugar. Its nutritional value is the same. Likewise, raw sugar is sucrose, just like white sugar. Raw sugar may be less refined than white sugar, but again this does not offer any nutritional advantage. Contrary to popular opinion, honey offers no special health benefits. It consists of two simple sugars, glucose and fructose, just like white sugar. Thus, the body uses honey the same way as it would white sugar. Honey contains only trace amounts of vitamins and minerals, and one would have to eat very large quantities before any nutritional benefit would be gained.

FRUCTOSE (OR HFCS): IS IT METABOLICALLY OR NUTRITIONALLY UNIQUE?

Fructose comes from three main sources:

1. *natural sources* such as fruits, some sweet vegetables, and honey

2. *sucrose*, or common table sugar (which is 50 percent fructose)

3. *high-fructose corn syrup* or HFCS (which is up to 55 percent fructose).

While some argue that the *addition* of fructose to foods and beverages is "natural" because fructose is found *naturally* in fruit and other foods, the clear difference is that the *quantity* of fructose that we get from fruit pales in comparison to the amount we get from processed foods. A second difference is that fructose in fruit serves as a "signal" for sweetness, energy, and nutrition. This sweet taste encouraged our ancestors to seek out fruit for both pleasure and good health. In contrast, when we consume processed and refined foods sweetened with HFCS, we get the sweetness and calories, but little else. We are essentially being short-changed on nutrients. But perhaps there could be other problems as well.

High-fructose corn syrup (HFCS) was first developed in the mid-1960s. It starts out as cornstarch, which is chemically or enzymatically degraded to glucose and

FRUCTOSE COMES FROM THREE MAIN SOURCES

• *Natural sources* such as fruits, some sweet vegetables and honey

• *Sucrose* or common table sugar (which is 50 percent fructose)

• *High-fructose corn syrup* or HFCS (which is made from corn starch and up to 55 percent fructose)

some short polymers of glucose. Another enzyme is then used to convert varying fractions of glucose into fructose. Because of its unique physical and functional properties (e.g., stability in acidic foods and beverages, such as soft drinks), it was widely embraced by food formulators. In fact, while the intake of certain refined sugars, such as cane sugar, has declined over the last 40 years, the amount of fructose (particularly in the form of HFCS) has increased dramatically, principally as an attractive replacement for table sugar.[79] Why? Mainly because it's super-sweet (about six times sweeter than cane sugar), it's cheap (effectively subsidized by the federal price supports for corn), and because it is liquid, meaning that it can easily be directly pumped into processed foods and drinks. Today, HFCS serves as a visible marker for foods that are highly processed and refined. According to the USDA, the average American consumes more than 40 pounds of high-fructose corn syrup per year.

Although HFCS is chemically similar to sucrose (though with a slightly higher percentage of fructose), concerns have been raised that our bodies may react differently to HFCS than they do to other types of sweeteners. As stated previously, research has linked the consumption of SSBs (which are typically sweetened with HFCS) with weight gain. But the real question is, are the adverse effects of excessive SSBs simply due to the fact that they contain "added sugars" (i.e., empty sugar calories)? Is it because they contain HFCS, or higher amounts of fructose, specifically? This is where the controversy lies.

On one hand, there is a body of research showing that a high intake of fructose, unlike other sugars, raises serum uric acid levels (see *Figure 8, page 83)*. Nakagawa and colleagues[80] proposed that this happens when fructose is metabolized in the liver, its major organ for metabolism. High levels of uric acid could set the stage for advancing cardiovascular disease by reducing the availability of nitric oxide. Nitric oxide is crucial for maintaining normal blood pressure and for maintaining normal function of the endothelium (the interior layer of all blood vessel walls). Indeed, one study,[81] based on NHANES data from over 4,500 adults, found that, after adjusting for potential confounding factors, those who reported eating or drinking 74 grams of fructose or more per day (the equivalent of 2.5 sugary soft drinks per day) had a higher risk of hypertension than those who consumed less. The authors theorized that HFCS raises uric acid levels, which then increases blood pressure. In other research, excessive fructose consumption alone, or from HFCS, has been linked to visceral adiposity (abdominal fat), insulin resistance, high triglycerides, and fatty liver disease, leading some experts to conclude that high amounts of fructose may play an important role in the current epidemics of obesity, diabetes, and cardiovascular disease.[54,58,71,82-86]

Other researchers, however, contend that such claims are untrue.[87-90] They assert that, from a *compositional* standpoint, HFCS, sucrose, honey, invert sugar, and concentrated fruit juices are identical and essentially interchangeable. All of these nutritive sweeteners are composed of approximately 50 percent glucose and 50 percent fructose (though the amount of fructose may be slightly higher in HFCS). All are absorbed similarly, have similar sweetness, and have the same number of calories per gram. They argue that, from a *metabolic* standpoint, there are no significant differences between HFCS and sucrose in terms of endocrine, hormonal, or appetitive responses to these sweeteners. One review[88] concluded that, despite the epidemiological parallel between fructose consumption and obesity, there is no **direct** evidence linking obesity to the consumption of physiological amounts of fructose in humans (100 grams or less per day). Moreover, the review concluded that a moderate dose (50 grams or less per day) of added fructose has no deleterious effect on fasting and postprandial triglycerides (blood fats), hypertension, glucose control, or insulin resistance.[88] While the review agreed that high fructose intake may induce high uric acid levels, they state this occurs mainly in patients with gout.[88] Another review[89] concluded that fructose does not cause biologically relevant changes in triglycerides or body weight when consumed at levels approaching the 95th percentile estimates of intake. In a third review,[90] researchers concluded that there is no unequivocal evidence that moderate fructose intake is directly related to adverse events in humans and that there is no direct evidence of more serious metabolic consequences of HFCS versus sucrose consumption.

However, one of the most recent studies,[91] a brain-imaging study of healthy volunteers, showed that fructose consumption actually promoted changes in the brain that contribute to overeating. The study provided evidence that fructose modulates neurobiological pathways involved in appetite regulation, resulting in increased food intake. Moreover, fructose consumption was associated with reduced systemic levels of insulin, a key satiety-signaling hormone in the brain. The lead author stated, "Advances in food processing and economic forces leading

Fructose effects in the brain may contribute to overeating.

to increased intake of added sugar and accompanying fructose in the U.S. diet are indeed extending the supersizing concept to the population's collective waistlines."

Perhaps another mechanism by which fructose could potentially contribute to weight gain, or to other metabolic effects, is by modulating gut microbes. Gut bacteria are sensitive to differences in diet. That's important because the profile of this bacteria, our microbiome, can significantly influence metabolism, energy yield from food, the regulation of fat storage, insulin sensitivity, and even inflammatory activity in the body.[92-93] New research suggests that fructose, in particular, can *condition* gut bacteria to acquire a more "westernized" microbiome, resulting in an unfavorable metabolic state.[94]

Clearly, more research is needed to fully understand the metabolic effect of dietary fructose in humans and to determine whether there are any unique attributes of fructose or HFCS that make it particularly problematic. Until we know more, it may be best to simply focus on reducing ALL added sugars from our diet, because the fact of the matter is that too much of *any* caloric sweetener can pose a problem (whether it's derived from corn,

> Research on fructose and HFCS continues to evolve. Until we know more, it may be best to simply focus on reducing ALL added sugars from our diet.

sugar cane, beets, or fruit juice concentrate). Excessive consumption of any source of sugar can promote weight gain and a range of metabolic abnormalities, and adverse health conditions, as well as shortfalls of essential nutrients.[54]

ADDED SUGARS/REFINED CARBOHYDRATES & MEMORY DECLINE

We are just beginning to appreciate the toll that high intake of sugars or refined carbohydrates is taking on our brains. Our brains need sugar/glucose to function. In fact, they need about twice the amount of other cells in the body. So you can think of sugar/glucose as the "gasoline" of the brain. But the problem is that when we are taking in a lot of *added* sugars/refined carbohydrates, it can be quite detrimental. For example, high glycemic load diets/meals have been shown to:

- impair short-term (post-meal) memory performance in humans, and to promote long-term memory impairment in animal models[95]

- promote post-meal spikes in blood glucose, which favor inflammation and a state of oxidative stress,[96]

- induce hypoglycemia (as a result of the rapid flux of glucose and insulin), which can trigger central stress axes—essentially putting the body into a state of stress or shock[97]

- promote peripheral insulin resistance and high triglycerides (both of which contribute to insulin resistance in the brain, thus preventing the brain from using glucose normally).

For all of the above reasons, a diet high in added sugars/refined carbohydrate is likely to be bad for the brain. This "brain drain" could ultimately contribute to cognitive decline. But it appears that the worst culprit may be excess fructose (HFCS). A diet high in fructose, in particular, is linked to peripheral insulin resistance and hyperinsulinemia (high blood insulin).[79] Chronic high blood insulin has been shown to disrupt normal insulin signaling or insulin action in the brain. That's important because insulin has a neurotrophic, or protective, effect on the brain, regulating and maintaining cognitive function.[98,99] Animal studies show that a diet high in fructose alters the brains ability to learn and remember information.[100] Moreover, a high-fructose diet is linked to high blood triglycerides. Insulin resistance and high blood triglycerides are key risk factors for cardiovascular disease,[79] which is important because there is a strong link heart disease and brain health—what's good for the heart is good for the brain.

> Poor quality carbs are a brain drain.

How to Reduce Added Sugar/Refined Carbohydrates in Your Diet

1. **Be a savvy consumer.**

   - *Read ingredient lists.* Ingredients must be listed in descending order by weight. So, if you see sugar listed among the first few ingredients, the product is likely to be high in added sugar. But be aware, a product can have several different kinds of sweeteners that are each listed separately. This label manipulation, known as "ingredient splitting," serves to push each sweetener further down the list. That way, for example, even though more than one third of the box may be added sugar, the word "sugar" doesn't have to appear toward the top of the ingredient list and the product *appears* healthier, with healthier ingredients now listed toward the top.

- *Know that sugars/sweeteners can go by many different names, depending on their source and how they are made.* Examples include barley malt, beet sugar, brown sugar, cane-juice crystals, cane sugar, caramel, carob syrup, corn syrup, corn syrup solids, date sugar, dextran, dextrose, diastatic malt, ethyl maltol, fructose, fruit juice, fruit juice concentrate, glucose/ glucose solids, golden sugar, grape sugar, high-fructose corn syrup, honey, invert sugar, lactose, malt syrup, maltodextrin, maltose, mannitol, molasses, raw sugar, refiner's syrup, sorbitol, sorghum syrup, sucrose, sugar, turbinado sugar.

- **_Read the Nutrition Facts label._** The label is required to list an item's _total_ sugar per serving. However, it does not have to distinguish between "added" sugar and naturally occurring sugar.

2. **Take a "sweet retreat." Lower the "sweet volume" to reduce your "sweet threshold."** The goal is to reawaken the body's ability to taste the subtle, _natural_ sweetness found in _real, whole_ foods. Allow your taste buds to become more sensitive to sugar(s), so that the foods you want to limit, such as SSBs, candy, cakes, and cookies, are simply less appealing.

- have fresh fruit for dessert instead of candy, cake, cookies, pie, or other sweets

- if you choose canned fruit, make sure it's packed in water or juice, not syrup; enjoy sweeter vegetables, such as sweet potatoes, and even green veggies, such as fresh snap peas

- snack on vegetables, fruit, low-fat cheese, whole-grain crackers, and low-fat, low-calorie yogurt instead of candy, pastries, and cookies

- choose breakfast cereals carefully; avoid those with a high amount of total sugar

- consume less processed foods that contain added sugar, such as honey-nut waffles

- be aware that processed milk products, such as sweetened yogurt, and dairy-based desserts, such as ice cream, can contain lots of added sugar

- go easy on the condiments—sugar is added to salad dressings and ketchup; choose low-sugar varieties of syrups, jams, jellies, and preserves

3. **Think before you drink.**

- *Drink more water, unsweetened coffee and tea, and nonfat milk.* Get your taste buds accustomed to consuming fluids that are not sweet. Remember, sugar sweetened beverages

(SSBs) are the **major** source of added sugars in our diets. By reducing our consumption of soft drinks, we can significantly decrease the amount of empty sugar calories we consume.

- *Drink fewer blended coffee drinks* that contain flavored syrup and sweet toppings.

- *Drink fewer fruit drinks and less fruit juice.* While fruit juice can provide some vitamins and nutrients, it often contains high amounts of sugar (even the 100 percent fruit juice varieties) and lots of calories. At the same time, fruit juices and drinks lack the fiber (which has a satiety effect) and phytochemicals found in whole fruit.

4. **Focus on QUALITY carbs—high fiber, low glycemic load, whole foods.** Fiber promotes satiety through a number of hormonal, intestinal, and intrinsic effects. In other words, fiber has "staying power." Research has shown that people who eat higher fiber meals, eat less at their next eating opportunity. A higher fiber diet can help

smooth out hormonal swings that otherwise might promote intense cravings and overeating. Aim for approximately 14 grams of dietary fiber for every 1,000 calories consumed. But rather than selecting processed foods that have fiber added to them, choose real, whole foods that are naturally rich in fiber.

Besides fiber, focus on consuming lower glycemic load carbs, the one's that will be digested and absorbed more slowly. In general, higher-fiber foods will be lower glycemic load carbs. Just like fiber, low glycemic load foods provide a much greater satiety effect. Why? Because they have a slower rate of absorption, low glycemic load carbs promote more stable blood sugar. High glycemic load foods, by contrast, are digested and absorbed more rapidly, causing rapid fluctuations in glucose and insulin levels, which can make your appetite go wild—as if they stoke that Tasmanian beast of an appetite inside!

Heroin is to methadone, as refined sugar is to a low glycemic load food.

Table 4. *Glycemic load of selected foods*

LOW GLYCEMIC LOAD (10 OR UNDER)	• High-fiber fruits and vegetables (not including potatoes) • Bran cereals (1 oz) • Many legumes, including chick peas, kidney beans, black beans, lentils, pinto beans (5 oz cooked, approx. 3/4 cup)
MEDIUM GLYCEMIC LOAD (11-19)	• Pearled barley: 1 cup cooked • Brown rice: 3/4 cup cooked • Oatmeal: 1 cup cooked • Bulgur: 3/4 cup cooked • Rice cakes: 3 cakes • Whole grain breads: 1 slice • Whole-grain pasta: 1¼ cup cooked
HIGH GLYCEMIC LOAD (20+)	• Baked potato , French fries • Refined breakfast cereal: 1 oz • Sugar-sweetened beverages: 12 oz • Jelly beans: 10 large or 30 small • Candy bars: 1 2-oz bar or 3 mini bars • Couscous: 1 cup cooked • Cranberry juice cocktail: 8 oz • White basmati rice: 1 cup cooked • White-flour pasta: 1¼ cup cooked

Some have likened the effect of low glycemic load foods methadone: *Heroin is to methadone as refined sugar is to a low glycemic load food.* Like methadone, low glycemic load foods enter the system more slowly and produce less compulsive intake. That makes them less seductive. Over the long term, low glycemic load foods can help with appetite regulation by improving insulin sensitivity, both peripherally and centrally (in the brain). Instead of promoting insulin surges, hyperinsulinemia and eventual insulin resistance, low glycemic load carbs cause a more gradual, gentle rise in blood glucose and insulin. I am convinced that reducing blood sugar volatility and improving insulin action (especially in the brain) is a key component of appetite control. *Table 4* lists some examples of low vs. high glycemic load foods. While it's good to know about fiber and glycemic load, the reality is that people probably really don't need to get bogged down by all this information if they follow one simple rule: EAT REAL, WHOLE FOODS!

Chapter 6

What About Sweetener Substitutes?

Based on what was discussed in **Chapter 5,** regarding the problems associated with consuming too much added sugars, you might think that you'd be better off with a sugar substitute instead. The rationale for using sweetener substitutes is that they can react with receptors on the tongue to give people the sensation of tasting something sweet without the calories associated with natural sweeteners, such as table sugar.

Sweetener substitutes can be classified in a number of different ways. One way is to group them according to the calories they provide, as being either "nutritive" (providing calories) or "non-nutritive" (not providing calories).[101] For example, sugar alcohols *(or **polyols**;*

see page 123) are considered to be nutritive sugar substitutes because they provide calories. However, they sweeten with only two calories per gram vs. the four calories per gram found in table sugar. Moreover, because they are not fully absorbed from the gut, sugar alcohols are less available for energy metabolism. Non-nutritive sweeteners, on the other hand, provide zero calories (or insignificant calories) and, because they sweeten with little volume, they can be referred to as high-intensity sweeteners. Because both nutritive and non-nutritive sweeteners can replace sugar sweeteners, they are referred to as *sugar substitutes, sugar replacers,* or *alternative sweeteners.*[101] The term "artificial" sweeteners is generally used for synthetic, non-nutritive sugar substitutes, though they may be derived from naturally-occurring substances as well.

Currently, the U.S. Food and Drug Administration (FDA) has approved five nonnutritive sweeteners for consumption—acesulfame potassium, aspartame, neotame, saccharin, and sucralose. *Table 5* lists the FDA's Acceptable Daily Intake (ADI) and the

Table 5. U.S. Food and Drug Administration-approved non-nutritive sweeteners

Name	Examples	Acceptable Daily Intake (per day)	Estimated Daily Intake (per day)
Acesulfame-K	Sunett®, Sweet One®	15 mg/kg body weight	3 mg/kg body weight
Aspartame (the "blue packet")	Equal®, NutraSweet®	50 mg/kg body weight	3 mg/kg body weight
Neotame (derived from aspartame)	Used in baked goods, soft drinks, chewing gum, frozen desserts	18 mg/kg body weight	0.04 mg/kg body weight
Saccharin (the "pink packet")	Sweet'N Low® SugarTwin®	15 mg/kg body weight	1.8 mg/kg body weight

Estimated Daily Intake (EDI) for each sweetener. The ADI is defined as the weight of sweetener (per kilogram of body weight) that a person can safely consume every day over a lifetime without apparent risk. This is considered to be conservative estimate that reflects 1/100 of the maximum level that presumably produces no adverse effects. The EDI is an estimate of the weight of sweetener consumed (per kilogram of body weight per day) based on food consumption surveys.

As can be seen in **Table 5**, the average estimated consumption of nonnutritive sweeteners (the EDI) is well below the ADI. For example, one packet of Equal contains 35 to 40 mg of aspartame, one 12-ounce diet soda contains 225 mg of aspartame, and one 8-ounce yogurt contains 80 mg of aspartame. Thus, a 150-pound adult would have to drink approximately 15 cans of diet soda sweetened with aspartame to exceed the ADI. Likewise, it would take five cans of Diet Coke sweetened with sucralose and 8.5 packets of saccharin, and 25 cans of Diet Coke containing acesulfame-K to reach the respective artificial-sweetener ADIs.

ARE THESE SWEETENERS HELPFUL FOR WEIGHT LOSS?

Over the past several decades, more and more people have been using artificial or non-nutritive sweeteners in an attempt to lose or control weight. Artificial sweeteners have been viewed as dietary tools that can help people adhere to their weight-loss plans. The widespread belief has been that these products are beneficial because they provide a sweet taste without the extra calories found in sugary foods and beverages. However, over the past few years, the metabolic health benefits of these products have come under scrutiny. Are these sweeteners truly helpful for weight loss or weight management? Is it really appropriate to advocate their use in place of sugar-sweetened products?

On one hand, some research has demonstrated beneficial effects of artificial sweeteners. For example, the Nurses' Health Study II, a prospective cohort study, found that adults who consumed artificially-sweetened beverages were less likely to gain weight.[102] Moreover, randomized controlled trials have shown a link between artificial sweetener use and weight stability or minimal short-term weight loss (compared with caloric sweeteners),[103,104] as well as decreased weight regain after dieting.[105] In contrast, an extensive review paper by Mattes[106] concluded that, while the use of artificial sweeteners may promote a reduction in calorie intake (of about 5 to 15 percent per day), there is little evidence that these products actually promote weight loss over the long term. This review determined that, unless there is calorie restriction, the addition of artificial sweeteners to diets poses no benefit for weight loss.

More recently, a few studies have suggested that these sweeteners might actually have an opposite effect, promoting detrimental effects on body weight. One example is a large scale prospective cohort study called the San Antonio Heart Study,[107] which followed more than 5,000 adults for seven to eight years. This study found that, after adjusting for confounding factors, those subjects who consumed the highest amount of artificial sweeteners actually gained more weight than those who consumed the least. They published their findings in paper entitled: "Fueling the obesity epidemic? Artificially-sweetened beverage use and long-term weight gain."[107] Other large, prospective cohort studies in adults have linked intake of artificial sweeteners with the incidence of metabolic syndrome and its components, including increased waist circumference, high blood pressure, and elevated fasting blood sugar.[108-111]

Epidemiologic studies conducted with children have shown a link between artificial sweetener intake (most commonly in the form of diet soda) and weight gain as well.[112] But, the few small, randomized, controlled trials conducted in children have not found an association between artificial sweetener consumption and weight change.[112]

Part of the difficulty in determining whether these products have detrimental effects is that sweetener intake is likely to serve as an indicator for other, potentially confounding, variables. For example, people often decide to switch to artificial sweeteners when they become concerned about their weight and want to reduce their calorie intake. Thus, the use of these sweeteners may simply serve as a "marker" for individuals who are already on weight-gain trajectories, which continue despite their switching to artificial sweeteners. Likewise, for children, the decision to use artificial sweeteners is often made by parents who are concerned about their own weight, and consequently the weight of their offspring, thus further confounding the choice to use artificial sweeteners with genetic and behavioral variables.[112]

If there is a positive association between nonnutritive sweeteners and weight gain, the question is why? Multiple mechanisms have been proposed:

- **The dissociation of the sensation of sweet taste from caloric intake may confuse the brain and disrupt appetite regulation.** One study that supports this contention is a rat study[113] in which the animals were fed either yogurt sweetened with glucose or saccharin, the oldest of all artificial sweeteners. The results showed that animals fed the saccharin-laced yogurt, ate more yogurt and gained more weight. Why? Here's one interpretation: in nature, a sweet taste is a good predictor of the caloric content of foods. Eating "real" sugar (sweetness + calories) sets off a response to let the body know that "real" calories are being consumed. In turn, the animal is satisfied. But if they eat a very sweet yogurt that is sweetened with an artificial sweetener, it's as if the body is searching for calories to match the sweet taste. And, as a result, the animal ends up consuming more (in this case, yogurt) to compensate—a phenomenon referred to as *physiological compensation*. So, from this perspective, I guess you could say: "You can't fool mother nature."

In recent review paper, Dr. Susan Swithers, a professor of behavioral neuroscience, asserts that frequent consumers of sugar substitutes may ultimately be at increased risk of excessive weight gain, metabolic syndrome, type 2 diabetes and cardiovascular disease, in part because such products "interfere with learned relationships between sweet taste and post-ingestive outcomes."[114] She suggests that this may, in turn, impair our ability to compensate for energy when caloric sweeteners are consumed. In other words, artificial sweeteners confuse the brain so that it can't tell when sweetness actually equals calories and, as a result, the normal regulation of appetite and energy balance may become disrupted.

> When it comes to sugar substitutes, it appears that *YOU JUST CAN'T FOOL MOTHER NATURE!*

- **Artificial sweeteners may alter taste preferences.** Aspartame, acesulfame potassium, saccharin, sucralose, and neotame are 180, 200, 300, 600, and 7,000 to 13,000 times sweeter than sugar, respectively. Some experts contend that the intense sweetness of these substances leads to taste distortion, essentially raising our "sweet threshold" and increasing our preference for sweet flavors overall.[107] We become "conditioned" to seek out sweet flavors. This is a concern because sweet-dependency ultimately drives many chronic diseases. This preference toward sweet flavors could stimulate our appetites[28] and reduce the quality of our diets overall.

- **Consumers use diet products as a rationale for consuming more high-calorie foods.**[107] Some experts suggest that consumers of "lite" products overestimate caloric savings achieved by using artificial sweeteners, and unintentionally overcompensate elsewhere in their diets. It's the "I'm having a diet soda, so I can have an extra slice of pecan pie," mentality. This is referred to as *psychological compensation*.

- **Artificial sweeteners have an effect on gut metabolism.** New data from both human and animal models have provided convincing evidence that artificial sweeteners play an active role in the gastrointestinal tract. They appear to be capable of activating receptors in the gut, thus influencing glucose absorption from the intestine into the blood stream.[115] They also appear to influence the secretion of gut hormones, which may potentially alter both gastric emptying and insulin secretion.[116-120]

- **Artificial sweeteners may modify how the body handles sugar.** In a study[121] of obese individuals given either water or sucralose (Splenda) prior to a glucose challenge test, it was shown that sucralose caused the blood sugar to peak at a higher level (as compared to water). Insulin levels also rose about 20 percent higher in the sucralose group, though the researchers do not know the mechanism responsible. Whether these acute effects will influence how our bodies handle sugar in the *long term* is still not known. However, if a person routinely secretes more and more insulin, over time they can become resistant to its effects, a path that can lead to the development of type 2 diabetes and other metabolic complications. Clearly, products such as sucralose are much more than just something sweet that you put into your mouth with no other consequences.

- **Artificial sweeteners may impact the gut microbiome.** Limited research suggests that nonnutritive sweeteners could affect the gut microbiota. This could influence our ability to extract calories from food, as well as trigger a chronic inflammatory process that has been associated with the development of metabolic disorders.[122]

- **Artificial sweeteners have a direct effect on the appetite control center of the brain (in animal models).** Rodent studies have shown that high levels of aspartate—which constitutes 40 percent of aspartame—are toxic to neurons in the arcuate nucleus of the hypothalamus,[123,124] a key forebrain site that is important for appetite regulation. These animal studies have shown that the earlier the exposure, especially in utero, the more profound the damage.[123,124] In fact, neonatal exposure by injection produced "...an almost total absence of neurons in the arcuate nucleus."[124] Such findings have caused some experts to question whether aspartame exposure at high levels could cause neurotoxicity in humans as well, but this is not known.

So what's the bottom line—should these sweeteners be recommended? At this point in time, we lack sufficient evidence to state with certainty that artificial sweeteners *cause* weight gain or any other adverse health effects. In 2012, the American Heart Association (AHA) and the American Diabetes Association (ADA) issued a joint scientific statement[125-126] cautiously recommending the use of nonnutritive sweeteners in order to help people maintain a healthy body weight, and to aid diabetics in glucose control. The statement says:

> There are some data to suggest that nonnutritive sweeteners may be used in a structured diet to replace sources of added sugars and that this substitution may result in modest energy-intake reductions, weight loss, and beneficial effects on related metabolic parameters.

However, the statement also says that, "Scientific evidence is limited and inconclusive about whether this strategy is effective in the *long run* for reducing calorie and added-sugars consumption." It stresses that such sweeteners are only helpful if people don't consume *additional* calories later, whether it be physiological or psychological compensation.

Are these artificial sweeteners safe? Are they preferable to sugar? The AHA/ADA statement (described above) did not pass any judgment on the safety of these substances. The National Cancer Institute and other health agencies have determined that there's no sound scientific evidence that any of these FDA-approved artificial sweeteners cause cancer or other serious health problems. But do keep in mind that having FDA approval is not necessarily a definitive indication of the products' safety. The reality is that very little is known about the health consequences of consuming artificial sweeteners over the course of a lifetime.[58] We simply cannot be completely sure about the long-term safety of these products. Dr. Paul Breslin, a researcher who studies taste perception, has said. "We won't know what the high-potency sweeteners in our diet are doing to us for another 40 or 50 years. Essentially it is a natural experiment on the population, and the jury is still out." Until we know more, it may be prudent to use such products *in moderation.* They should not be viewed as a magic bullet for weight loss. And it is important to consider that most products that contain these sweeteners generally don't offer the same health benefits as do whole foods, such as fruits and vegetables.

> "We won't know what the high-potency sweeteners in our diet are doing to us for another 40 or 50 years. Essentially it is a natural experiment on the population, and the jury is still out."

Perhaps a more pertinent question is: Are nonnutritive sweeteners a better alternative than sugar? Most experts would agree that the artificial sweeteners on the market are safer than consuming large amounts of regular sugar. As stated previously, high consumption of sugar, especially when consumed in beverage form such as soda, has been shown to increase the risk of obesity, diabetes, cardiovascular disease, and other health problems. However, a real concern is that just replacing sugar with artificial sweeteners can condition people, particularly children, to high levels of sweetness or, in other words, raise their sweet threshold. This, in turn, is likely to adversely influence their food choices. Dr. Walter Willett of Harvard School of Public Health has suggested that we consider these products to be like a nicotine patch; they are appreciably better than the real product (sugar), but not part of an optimal diet. So for those who want to kick the habit of drinking sugary soda, diet soda could be used in small amounts, for a short period of time (like a nicotine patch). But for most people, plain water and unsweetened coffee or tea are much more healthy alternatives that sugar-sweetened or diet sodas.

"We should consider artificial sweeteners to be like a nicotine patch; they are appreciably better than the real product (sugar), but not part of an optimal diet."

OTHER SUGAR SUBSTITUTES

Sugar alcohols (polyols). Sugar alcohols are carbohydrates that occur naturally in certain fruits and vegetables, but they can also be manufactured. Approved sugar alcohols include: erythritol, lactitol, maltitol, mannitol, sorbitol, and xylitol.

Possible Benefits:

- *weight control.* Sugar alcohols are considered to be nutritive sweeteners because they contribute calories to your diet, but because they are not completely absorbed in the intestine, they contain two calories per gram vs. four calories per gram for sucrose)

- *diabetes.* Unlike artificial sweeteners, sugar alcohols can raise blood sugar levels because they're carbohydrates. But they produce less of a glycemic response than table sugar

- *dental cavities.* Sugar alcohols don't promote cavities. In fact, use of polyol-based gums (especially xylitol) may actually *reduce* the risk of dental caries[101]

Disadavantages:

- not noncaloric (but lower in calories than sugar)

- Sugar alcohols can have a laxative effect, causing bloating, intestinal gas, and diarrhea if consumed in large amounts (which can be as much as 50 grams per day, or as little as 10 grams, depending on the individual)

"Natural" sweeteners. Natural sweeteners (such as date sugar, grape juice concentrate, honey, maple syrup, molasses, and agave nectar) are sugar alternatives that are often touted as *healthier* options than processed table sugar or artificial sweeteners. Despite the claims that these sweeteners are more *"natural,"* they often undergo at least some processing and refining. Moreover, their vitamin and mineral content isn't significantly different from that of table sugar; they contain the same amount of calories. And natural sweeteners can raise your blood sugar, just as table sugar can. However, agave nectar (which is composed predominantly of fructose), does have a lower glycemic load than table sugar[127] and, therefore,

presumably don't cause blood sugar to rise as quickly as other sweeteners. Finally, natural sweeteners can contribute to tooth decay. The general consensus is that there is no significant benefit to using these instead of regular table sugar.

Stevia. *Stevia rebaudiana* is a South American shrub in the chrysanthemum family whose leaves have been used for centuries by people in Paraguay, Argentina, and Brazil to sweeten beverages. The sweetness of these leaves is the result of a mixture of chemicals called steviol glycosides (SGs). Currently, the FDA does not permit the use of crude whole-leaf extracts of stevia in conventional foods because of safety concerns, though it can be sold as a dietary supplement. Animal studies have suggested that crude or partially purified stevia leaf extracts are linked to adverse renal, cardiovascular and particularly reproductive effects. Interestingly, Guarani Indians in Paraguay traditionally consumed a decoction of the leaf extracts as an oral contraceptive. On the other hand, studies conducted with preparations of the SGs themselves, (e.g., stevioside, rebaudioside A) have shown no adverse effects. In December of 2008, the FDA added the highly refined stevia leaf extract to its list of GRAS (Generally Regarded as Safe) substances, thus giving it the "green light" to be incorporated into foods. A Joint Food and Agriculture Organization/World Health Organization Expert Committee on Food Additives established an acceptable daily intake for SGs as 0 to 4 mg per kg body weight (expressed as steviol equivalents).[128] Stevioside (also known as rebaudioside A or rebiana) is one of the SGs that has been extracted from the plant. Truvia™ is one of the consumer products that contains rebiana marketed by Cargill and developed jointly with the Coca-Cola Company; Pure Via™ is another rebiana product marketed by The Merisant Company (maker of Equal®) and the PepsiCo brand. These products are sold both as tabletop sweeteners and as ingredients in a wide range of sweetened products, including beverages.

Rebiana has no calories and is about 250 to 300 times sweeter than sucrose (table sugar).[129] It has a negligible effect on blood sugar and tastes like sugar (while the whole leaf has a bitter or licorice-like aftertaste, refined versions are much closer in taste to sugar). Food companies have taken advantage of the fact that rebiana is derived from a plant; they can market it as a natural alternative to artificial sweeteners (though there is no specific definition for "natural"). There are many questions about whether this product deserves to wear its "natural halo" when it fact it is really a purified plant extract that is a far reach from how stevia appears in nature. Others are skeptical of the product, worried that consumers, dazzled by "green-leaf" marketing, wrongly perceive it as a healthy alternative to sugar. There is also concern that this intense sweetener (some 300 times sweeter than table sugar) has the potential to alter our food preferences. And we really don't know what effect it might have on our bodies, brains, and taste buds over the long term.

The bottom line is moderation. If you consume a few products sweetened by stevia extract on a daily basis, it is likely to pose no problem. However, consumers must keep in mind that just because something is *natural,* it does not necessarily always mean that it's safe if consumed in large quantities.

Chapter 7

Dietary Fats

When people think of fat, they think of body fat. That dietary fat makes you fat. That it is the major culprit in the battle against the bulge. Well, fat is a major source of fuel energy for the body. In fact, it packs in more than twice the caloric load of either carbohydrate or protein, at 9 calories per gram (vs. 4 calories for carbs and protein). But it also aids in the absorption of fat-soluble vitamins (vitamins A, D, E, and K) and phytochemicals, such as beta-carotene. And it is a major constituent of your brain. Your brain is approximately 60 percent fat by weight (we are fat-heads!). But, as we'll see later, the *types* of fats you eat can strongly influence brain function. Dietary fat is also important for maintaining the integrity of skin and cell membranes, and synthesizing important chemicals, such as prostaglandins and leukotrienes.

The food industry loves dietary fat because it gives baked foods more bulk and a firmer texture. It also extends the shelf-life, so processed food products can remain on your grocery shelf for months at a time. But perhaps far more important than these roles is the simple fact that fat makes food more desirable. It promotes the release of fat-enhancing chemicals, allowing flavors to merge and meld.

Interestingly, however, it appears that we cannot taste fat directly. That is, the taste of fat is not part of our official roster of primary tastes (sweet, salty, sour, bitter, and a more recent addition called umami, a meaty, savory taste derived from the amino acid glutamine). In fact, while all the other tastes have receptors in our taste buds that provide a vehicle to deliver that taste message to the brain, no such receptor has yet been identified for fat.[1] So, why then are we so drawn to it? Fat is all about "mouthfeel," that gooey, creamy, smooth sensation. And it's about texture, that crispy, crunchy experience. In fact, neurological science suggests that we are actually capable of feeling fat by way of the trigeminal nerve (the largest of the cranial nerves), which hovers above and behind the mouth, near the brain. This nerve has branches that are able to extract tactile information from the lips, gums, teeth, and jaw, and then convey that message of pleasure to the brain.[1] And, it is indeed an apparently very powerful message that draws us in to eat more.

The food industry views fat as a potent component of processed foods, a pillar ingredient that is perhaps even more powerful than sugar.[1] However, it seems that fat may have an advantage over sugar. Michael Moss's investigations[1] have discovered that fat doesn't blast away at our mouths like sugar does; it's allure is more secretive. No wonder that "binge" foods are so often high in fat, often combined with sugar, a combination that makes foods, such as high-fat ice cream or fudge brownies, so hyperpalatable that they seem simply irresistible.[26] Years ago, food companies discovered that there is essentially no limit to the bliss point for fat. They could add more and more to their products, and people would go crazy for it. That is, unless, consumers actually paid attention to the nutrition facts panel and discovered just how many calories a serving contained. It's that combination, a desirable mouthfeel or texture coupled with a dense source of calories that make dietary fat in processed foods so problematic from an obesity standpoint.

It appears, however, that the experience of fat goes way beyond the mouthfeel. In fact, new research suggests that fat can modulate our emotions *even if we can't taste it, or don't even know are consuming it.* In a very unique study,[130] subjects were randomized to be "fed," via an intragastric feeding tube, with either a blend of fatty acids or saline. Because the tubes were unmarked, subjects had no taste, sight, smell, or texture associated with what was being placed in the tube (i.e., they had no idea what was being funneled into their guts). The subjects were then further subdivided to listen to either neutral (classical) music or sad music (coupled with images of sad faces), while undergoing a functional MRI (fMRI). Interestingly, the brain scans showed that, compared to saline solution, subjects receiving the fatty solution (via the feeding tube) had dampened activity in parts of the brain that are involved in sadness and that respond to sad music/faces. Importantly, the fatty solution reduced the intensity of the sad emotions by almost half—which is clinically meaningful, since it is in the order of magnitude achieved by antidepressant medications. These results show that the effect of food on mood (or in this case, dietary fat on mood) can actually be *independent* of taste (or pleasant stimuli). This finding may provide a neurobiological explanation for well-known clinical phenomena, such as "emotional overeating," "comfort feeding," or appetite disturbances that are associated with mood disorders.[130,131]

> MRI scans show that fat modulates emotions, thus providing a neurobioogical explanation for "emotional overeating" or "comfort feeding."

Many people consider themselves to be "addicted" to fatty foods. However, this concept is not well understood, and it appears that not all palatable foods are similar in their effect on the expression of behaviors common to addiction. For example, in a study[132] of rats fed a fat-rich diet, withdrawal from fat did not result in opiate-like withdrawal symptoms, either when precipitated by the opiate antagonist naloxone or upon fasting, as has been previously shown with sugar.[133-134] Thus, while fat-rich foods may impart addiction-like effects, the lack of opiate-like withdrawal suggests that brain opioid systems are *differentially* affected by overeating fat-rich foods compared to overeating sugar.[8] Some experts suggest that while it is the fat that promotes the weight gain, it likely the sugar (or sweet taste) that is largely responsible for producing addictive-like behaviors (e.g., a withdrawal syndrome) in susceptible individuals who consume a diet high in poor quality, high-fat, high-sugar foods.[26]

"Official" recommendations for amount of fat to consume (as a percentage of total calories). The Dietary Guidelines for Americans[55] from the U.S. Department of Health and Human Services has established the following acceptable daily ranges for *total fat intake* for children and adults:

- **children ages 1 to 3 years** – 30 to 40 percent of total calories

- **children and adolescents ages 4 to 18 years** – 25 to 35 percent

- **adults ages 19 years and older** – 20 to 35 percent

However, we now understand that the *types* of fatty acids we consume are likely far more important in terms of influencing our risk for chronic disease than is the *total* amount of fat that we consume.

> The types of fatty acids we consume are likely far more important in terms of influencing our risk for chronic disease than is the total amount of fat we consume.

CLASSIFICATION OF DIETARY FATS

The fats in our diet contain a mixture of different kinds of fatty acids. Fatty acids vary in carbon chain length and degree of unsaturation (number of double bonds in the carbon chain). They can be classified as saturated, monounsaturated, or polyunsaturated *(see Figure 9)*. Saturated fatty acids are those that have

Figure 9. Classification of fatty acids

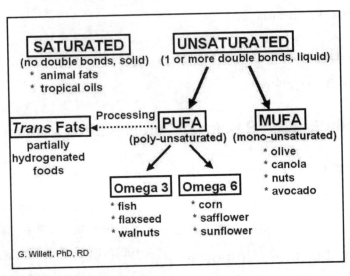

G. Willett, PhD, RD

no double bonds. Most fats with a high percentage of saturated fatty acids are solid at room temperature, such as animal fats and tropical oils, and are therefore referred to as "solid fats." Unsaturated fatty acids are those that have at least one or more double bonds, which makes them liquid at room temperature. They are referred to as "oils." Unsaturated fatty acids can be subdivided into monounsaturated fatty acids, which have one double bond, and polyunsaturated fatty acids, which have two or more double bonds. Within the category of polyunsaturated fats, there are the omega-3 fatty acids and the omega-6 fatty acids (see *Figure 9* for foods rich in these types of fatty acids). Finally, if a polyunsaturated fatty acid undergoes processing (is partially hydrogenated), it can convert to a *trans* fatty acid. This means that the adjacent hydrogen atoms are bound to *opposite* sides of the carbon-carbon double bond, causing the fatty acid chain to be straighter in shape, similar to saturated fatty acids (such differences in geometry play an important role in biological processes, and in the construction of biological structures such as cell membranes). *Trans*-fats are used because they are easier to cook with and less likely to spoil. But they have physical properties that generally resemble saturated fats. *Trans* are solid at room temperature, and, thus, are put in the category of "solid fats" *(see section, "Solid Fats," page 166)* In general, animal fats tend to have a higher proportion of saturated fatty acids (except for seafood) and plant foods tend to have a higher proportion of monounsaturated and/ or polyunsaturated fatty acids (except for tropical oils such as palm and palm kernel oil).

So Which Fats Should We limit?

Saturated Fatty Acids (SFAs)

The body uses some saturated fatty acids for physiological and structural functions, but it is capable of making more than enough to meet those needs. Therefore, humans have no dietary requirement for saturated fatty acids.[55]

Potential Health Concerns

1. **Heart disease.** In 1985, the National Heart, Lung, and Blood Institute launched the National Cholesterol Education Program (NCEP) with the goal of reducing illness and death from coronary heart disease in the United States by reducing the percent of Americans with high blood cholesterol. Over the years, a primary focus of their educational campaign has been to lower dietary SFA and cholesterol so as to improve blood lipid levels. Likewise, the American Heart Association promotes a low SFA diet to improve blood lipids and reduce heart disease risk. However, while evidence has linked consumption of SFA to

increased LDL-C levels (the "bad" cholesterol) and an increased risk of the development of cardiovascular disease (CVD), recent findings have indicated that the link between SFA and cardiovascular disease may be far less straightforward than originally thought.[135] A recent review paper[136] concluded that "the influence of dietary fats on serum cholesterol has been overstated." It contends that it is likely that *other* factors, such as oxidized polyunsaturated fatty acids (PUFAs) or preservatives found in highly processed meats—factors that are *also* present in high-SFA foods—are likely responsible for the adverse health effects typically associated with high SFA intake. This viewpoint remains controversial. Even if SFA do raise blood cholesterol levels, some researchers are now questioning whether that necessarily translates to higher heart disease risk. And a recent meta-analysis[137] of 21 prospective epidemiologic studies showed that

> Recent findings have indicated that the link between dietary SFA and CVD may be far less straightforward than originally thought.

there is insufficient evidence from prospective epidemiologic studies to conclude that *all* dietary SFA fat is necessarily associated with an increased risk of coronary heart disease, stroke, or CVD. Perhaps the *type* of SFA or the *food source* of SFA influences the health consequences associated with its consumption. The debate continues.

2. **Insulin resistance/diabetes.** Some research suggests that SFA may also increase the risk of type 2 diabetes because it promotes a state of insulin resistance.[138,139] And there is evidence that SFA can contribute to leptin resistance as well.[140] Both leptin (made by fat cells) and insulin (made by the pancreas) are key hormones important in the normal regulation of appetite, food intake, and body weight *(see **Figure 10**)*. Normally, when the amount of body fat increases, blood levels of both leptin and insulin also go up. These hormones then cross the blood-brain barrier to inform the brain of the level of fuel available to the body. As long as the brain can correctly interpret these signals, it will decrease the drive to eat and rev-up

Figure 10. *Saturated fat and dysregulation of body weight*

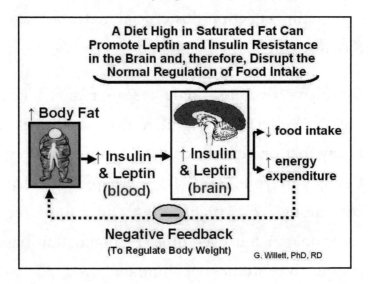

metabolism *(see **Figure 10**)*. However, if there is leptin and insulin resistance in the brain (i.e., the brain cannot accurately detect the signals), it may lead to a dysregulation of appetite and body weight regulation, and, as a result, weight gain.[141]

Animal research suggests that a high-fat diet can directly inflict damage to the hypothalamus,[42] the energy regulator of the brain, thus disrupting the normal nutrient-sensing and energy balance functions of the hypothalamus. This problem appears to be due, at least in part, to fat-induced hypothalamic inflammation, which has a debilitating effect on this crucial metabolic sensor. *(See discussion on inflammation, page 144)*

3. **Cognitive decline.** Some research has linked a high SFA diet with cognitive decline. This is not to say that one cheese danish is gonna tazer every thought in your head! But perhaps a *pattern* of consuming a diet high in SFA and refined sugars could take a toll over time. In population-based, prospective studies of humans aged 65 years and older, high intakes of SFA, but not *total* fat, consumed over a four- to six-year period, led to a greater risk for the development of Alzheimer's disease and myocardial infarctions.[142-143] It is proposed that high SFA intake could potentially alter cognitive function by promoting insulin resistance and/or elevating brain inflammation. Animals consuming diets high in SFA have elevated markers of brain or neuro-inflammation, which is associated with cognitive decline. They also have impaired spatial memory and reduced brain-derived neurotrophic factor, a protective

brain protein.[144] New research in humans suggests that SFA may make the brain more vulnerable to Alzheimer's disease. In a recent, small, randomized control trial,[145] cognitively normal subjects and subjects with mild cognitive impairment were randomized to consume calorie-equivalent diets characterized either as "Western" diets, ones high in SFA and refined carbohydrates (e.g., a typical meal consisting of cheeseburgers, fries, and sodas) or healthier diets, low in SFA and refined carbohydrates (e.g., a typical meal consisting of poached fish, brown rice, and steamed vegetables). After four weeks, it was shown the group consuming the Western diet high in SFA had more beta-amyloid plaque (a factor believed to contribute to Alzheimer's disease), in a toxic form that is more difficult to clear from the brain. They also had lower levels of insulin in their cerebral spinal fluid, suggesting that the Western diet decreased insulin transport into (or insulin activity within) the brain. This is important because insulin functions as a key neuropeptide.

4. **Chronic systemic inflammation.** Research suggests that a high-fat diet, but a high SFA diet in particular, is capable of activating the inflammasome *(see Figure 11).*[146,147] The inflammasome is a group of protein complexes that are an integral part of our body's immune system. You can think of them as special "danger sensing" proteins that are activated by bacteria, viruses, and other potentially harmful substances. Well, it turns out that a high SFA diet, and perhaps a poor quality, processed diet, in general, is capable of activating the inflammasome. One mechanism that may be involved is that certain dietary factors are capable of promoting a change in our gut bacteria which, in turn, activates the inflammasome. This is a concern because once the inflammasome is activated, it releases a whole host of inflammatory mediators that promote intestinal inflammation which, in turn, can promote systemic inflammation. Chronic systemic inflammation favors a state of insulin resistance. As tissues such as the liver, fat, and muscle become "blind" to insulin, it puts people at risk for type 2

Figure 11. *The proposed link between diet, inflammasome, and disease*

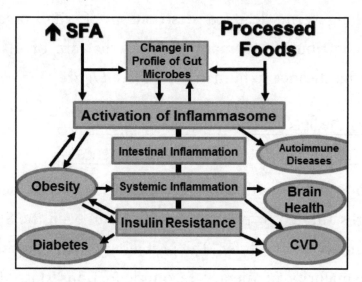

diabetes and cardiovascular disease. Moreover, chronic systemic inflammation is believed to, ultimately, contribute to brain inflammation, which could impact virtually every brain function relevant to health and behavior. Research suggests that activation of the inflammasome is a crucial step on the road from obesity to insulin resistance and type 2 diabetes.[148] And the inflammasome is critical for regulating the innate and adaptive immune responses. Aberrant activity could thus contribute to a range of autoinflammatory disorders and immune diseases. Thus, unchecked activation of the inflammasome could, over the long term, lead to destruction of vital organs contributing to many diseases that are of major significance to human health *(see **Figure 11**).*[149,150]

Does the Specific **Type** (or Chain Length) of Source of a Saturated Fat Make a Difference?

Foods are a mixture of different types of fatty acids (e.g. saturated or polyunsaturated). But even the SFA, themselves, can differ. The problem is that, currently, the majority of dietary recommendations state that we should reduce saturated fats, in general, in order to reduce risk of CVD (and other health outcomes), without taking into consideration the *specific* SFA, or food *source*.

In a typical Western diet, the majority of dietary SFAs consist of 12:0, 14:0, 16:0, and 18:0, meaning 12–18 carbons in the chain with 0 double bonds. However, the reality is that the SFA of different chain lengths may very well display different metabolic properties,[151] meaning that not all SFA are necessarily detrimental. For example, it appears that the tendency to elevate LDL-cholesterol (the "bad" cholesterol) and the tendency to promote insulin-resistance and diabetes may differ among individual SFA. Moreover, some individual SFA, when considered separately, may actually have some beneficial health effects. For instance, lauric acid (C12:0) and myristic acid (C14:0), have a greater total cholesterol raising effect than palmitic acid (C16:0). Stearic acid (C18:0), on the other hand, has a neutral effect on the concentration of *total* serum cholesterol, including no apparent impact on either LDL ("bad") or HDL ("good") cholesterol. Lauric acid has been shown to raise total serum cholesterol; however, it also raises HDL cholesterol.[152-154] Thus, clearly, to regard SFA as a single, homogenous group has probably been too much of an oversimplification. However, the problem is that, unfortunately, the role of *individual* SFA in metabolic disease is still poorly understood.[151] Therefore, based on the currently available evidence, it is simply not possible to give dietary recommendations based solely on the content of *individual* SFA.

> Clearly, to regard SFA as a single, homogenous group has probably been too much of an oversimplification.

Further complicating the picture, many foods that are considered to be high in SFA actually contain a wide array of *different* saturated and unsaturated fatty acids, each of which may differentially affect lipoprotein metabolism. Plus, these food sources also may contribute significant amounts of *other* nutrients, other phytochemicals, that may impact disease risk.[155] No wonder so many people, myself included, feel confused! To have a better understanding and to guide more precise dietary recommendations, we need more strictly controlled, short-term and long-term intervention studies that emphasize the differences between different SFA, food sources, origins, and foodstuffs. And, unfortunately, we're just not there yet.

Coconut oil. Coconut oil actually contains a higher percentage of saturated fat than most other fats or oil (including butter and lard). But if you turn on the TV, or surf the internet, you'd think it had superpowers. You hear internet entrepreneurs refer to its benefits as "near miraculous!" and that coconut oil can "melt away excess body fat," "protect against cancer," and even "cure Alzheimer's disease." Yet it is a highly saturated fat. Feel confused? You're not alone!

Coconut oil is obtained from the kernel of the coconut palm *(Cocos nucifera)*. What is unique about coconut oil is that most of its fatty acids are medium-chain fatty acids (predominately lauric acid, but also caprylic, myristic, and palmitic acids), as opposed to long-chain fatty acids (LCTs). Medium-chain triglycerides (MCTs) are the esterified form of medium-chain fatty acids; the terms are often used interchangeably. This may make a difference because our bodies metabolize MCTs differently than LCTs. For example, MCTs are rapidly metabolized, in the liver, into energy, and do not participate in the biosynthesis and transport of cholesterol. Thus, while we typically say that SFA raise cholesterol, this may not apply to *all foods* rich in SFAs. For example, in a small, short-term study[156] of Filipino women (age 35 to 69 years) examining the link between intake of coconut oil and blood lipids, coconut oil was not shown to elevate total cholesterol (TC), triglyceride levels, or the TC/HDL ratio, even after menopausal status was accounted for. In fact, coconut oil was associated with an increase in HDL-C ("good" cholesterol), perhaps because of its high lauric acid (12:0) content. In fact, coconut oil has a higher percentage of lauric acid than most other oils, which may be responsible for the unusual HDL-raising effects of coconut oil. This may explain why studies on Pacific Islanders, who have coconut as their staple food, have traditionally been shown to have a rather low incidence of CVD,[157] and studies in Sri-Lanka have shown that consumption of coconut is not associated with CVD in that population.[158] However, it's quite possible that something *else* about the diets, or physical activity, or genes of these populations could be responsible for neutralizing the potential rise in cholesterol from coconut oil use. Also, keep in mind that plant-based oils are more than just fats. They contain many antioxidants and other substances, so their overall effects on health can't be predicted simply by examining changes in LDL and HDL.

Some have argued that perhaps it's the *form* of coconut oil (virgin vs. conventional) that makes a difference in terms of heart disease risk. *Conventional* coconut oil—the kind used in some candies, coffee creamers, and movie theater popcorn—is made from dried coconut that is pulverized, cooked, and treated with chemicals to produce a bleached, refined oil for use in foods, whereas *virgin* coconut oil is made with a mild extraction procedure from fresh coconut meat. But the reality is that both virgin and conventional coconut oils contain the same SFA profile. And, unfortunately, studies looking at the effect of coconut oil—virgin or conventional—on heart disease in humans are scarce. The Center for Science in the Public Interest states that there is no good evidence that "virgin" coconut oil is any healthier than conventional coconut oil. Most experts recommend that coconut oil be used sparingly, primarily because the majority of the research to date has consisted of short-term studies specifically examining its effect on cholesterol levels. It may be that coconut oil's special HDL-boosting effect may make it "less bad" than its high saturated fat content would indicate, but it's still probably not the best choice among the many available oils, such as olive oil, to reduce the risk of heart disease.

What about the weight loss claims? As stated, coconut oil is a rich source of medium-chain triglycerides (MCTs). MCTs are rapidly metabolized, with less being stored in the fat tissue, thus suggesting a possible benefit for weight control. In a review[159] of 14 controlled clinical studies that used MCTs for weight loss, only one showed that MCTs were linked to an increase in satiety, and four showed an increase in energy expenditure. Thus, it was determined that, "the results are inconclusive and further controlled studies (with standardized amounts of MCT) are needed to determine if MCT can be recommended as alternative for obesity nutritional treatment." Since coconut oil contains only about half as much MCTs as actual MCT oil, it is not likely to have much more than a modest effect, if any. According to the Center for Science in the Public Interest: "there is no good evidence that coconut oil can help you lose weight."

Certainly, it is not likely to live up to the internet promises that it will "slim your waistline in a week."

Coconut oil is also being promoted to cure or prevent Alzheimer's disease. One major advocate is Dr. Mary Newport.[160] In 2003, her 53-year-old husband, Steve, started showing signs of dementia, which was later diagnosed as Alzheimer's disease (AD). She did some research and discovered that brain cells of patients with AD may have a hard time using glucose as an energy source (it's sometimes referred to as "diabetes of the brain", or "type 3" diabetes), but they can use ketones as an alternative fuel source, and coconut oil produces at least some ketones in the body. So she started giving her husband coconut oil and claimed that he made dramatic improvements. While that's certainly interesting anecdotal information, where' the science? The problem is that, while coconut oil does yield ketones, it takes a leap of faith to think that coconut oil would yield enough ketones to have a meaningful and persistent effect on Alzheimer's disease.[161] Still, some speculate that ketogenesis might improve free radical-medical pathologies

> Can coconut oil prevent heart disease, help you lose weight or protect the brain? Unfortunately, there's no good evidence that it does.

associated with AD.[162] According to the Alzheimer's Association, coconut oil should not be recommended for AD due to a lack of credible research evidence supporting efficacy. According to the Center for Science in the Public Interest, "there is no good evidence that coconut oil can cure Alzheimer's disease."

Dairy foods and dairy fat. Approximately two thirds of the fat in dairy fat is SFA, with the majority in the chain-length range of 4:0 to 18:0. Most health organizations state that, because of their high SFA content, high-fat dairy products (e.g., butter and whole milk) should be considered as a "less than optimal" food choices, especially in terms of reducing cardiovascular risk.[151] While there is strong evidence from short-term feeding studies to suggest that replacing dairy fat with unsaturated vegetable fat (e.g., canola oil) improves total and LDL-cholesterol,[163] other short-term intervention studies have shown that a diet higher in SFA, from whole milk and butter, may actually *increase* the HDL-cholesterol (the "good" cholesterol) when substituted for carbohydrates or unsaturated fatty acids.[164] So if dairy fat increases artery-clogging cholesterol, but also raises the protective kind of cholesterol, then perhaps it may be somewhat of a wash when it comes to blood lipids. The reality is that the majority of observational epidemiologic studies have failed to find an association between the intake of dairy products and increased risk of CVD, coronary heart disease, and stroke, *regardless* of milk fat levels.[164]

A systemic literature review[165] of observational studies examining the relationship between dairy fat and cardiometabolic disease determined that the evidence does *not* support the hypothesis that dairy fat or high-fat dairy foods contribute to obesity or cardiometabolic risk. In fact, it suggested that high-fat dairy consumption, within typical dietary patterns, is actually *inversely* associated with obesity risk, meaning that it protects against weight gain. Perhaps part of the explanation for this finding could be that fat has an important satiety effect—that "less fat" often makes you feel "less full." This may be the case, particularly in children. If a child drinks low-fat milk, but then grabs an extra cookie because of lingering hunger pangs, he or she may risk weight gain.

Nevertheless, *lower*-fat dairy products are still commonly recommended as part of a healthy diet, such as in the DASH (Dietary Approaches to Stop Hypertension) diet, which also promotes eating lots of fruit and vegetables, whole grains, nuts, legumes, and is low in processed and red meats, sweets, and salt.[151] This recommendation is based on data indicating that low-fat dairy foods can decrease blood pressure.[166] Low-fat dairy products are also a component of several dietary patterns that, as a whole, are associated with reduced mortality and cardiovascular risk. But the question is, Why? Perhaps it has nothing to do with the fat at all! While the mechanisms for the possible beneficial effects of low-fat dairy products are not well established, one explanation is that the calcium and vitamin D present in these foods may regulate fat cell metabolism and reduce body weight.[167]

Another explanation is that dietary calcium and whey in milk could affect the absorption and/or excretion of intestinal fatty acids and bile acids.[167-168]

Yes, it's confusing!! To further complicate the picture, it appears that *different* dairy products may also exert different effects. For instance, cheese has a lesser cholesterol-raising effect than butter, even if it has an equivalent milk fat content.[169] Cheese has even been suggested to have an overall *neutral* effect on CHD risk,[164,169] although evidence is limited. Since the fatty acid compositions among different dairy products are quite similar, it could be that *other* components of these foods, or other factors (e.g. fermentation) might explain these differing metabolic effects.[151]

Some researchers have questioned whether full-fat dairy products will have different effects depending upon whether the cows are free-range (grazing cows) versus conventionally fed (feed-lot) cows—the thought being that dairy products from grazing cows would have higher levels of, for example, bioactive components, derived from grass. In a double-blind, randomized, 12-week, parallel intervention study,[170]

38 healthy subjects replaced part of their habitual dietary fat intake with 39 grams of fat from test butter made from milk from mountain-pasture grazing cows or from cows fed conventional winter fodder. The result? No differences were observed in the two groups with regard to blood lipids or inflammatory markers. The authors concluded that dairy products from mountain-pasture grazing cows are not healthier than products from cows that are fed from high-input conventional systems.

The U.S. dairy industry made the "Got Milk?" slogan one of the all-time most famous slogans. And, over the years, the USDA and American Academy of Pediatrics have embraced it, recommending that all calorie-containing beverages be limited in the diet, except for low-fat milk. But now some experts are starting to have second thoughts. In their recent article[171] in *JAMA Pediatrics*, Dr. David Ludwig and Dr. Walter Willett questioned the scientific rationale for promoting reduced-fat milk consumption in children and adults (3 cups a day for most people), suggesting that we reconsider the role of cow's milk in human nutrition.[172] Besides addressing issues such as the greater satiety-effect of higher fat foods, and the mixed effect on dairy products on blood lipids, they questioned cow's milk consumption from an evolutionary perspective. They argue that grazing animals evolved to supply milk to their young, keeping them as close as possible in order to protect against predators. But as soon as calves turn into cows, and kids turn into goats, they stop drinking their mother's milk. So the question is, should adult humans continue to consume milk, especially from *another* animal? They also point to a hormone called insulin-like growth factor 1, found in milk products, that has been hypothesized to be linked to prostate and other cancers.[172]

So, should we drink cow's milk? This is an area which is being hotly debated. But, you may ask, if we cut out the milk, where are we going to get the calcium? What many people may not know is that you can easily meet your daily calcium requirements by eating leafy greens, nuts, and seeds. Almond and soy milk are favorite alternatives in my house.

Major sources of SFA in the U.S. diet. According to the 2010 Dietary Guidelines for Americans, the major sources of saturated fatty acids in the American diet (as a percentage of total SFA intake) include: regular (full-fat) cheese (account for about 9 percent of total saturated fat intake); pizza (6 percent); grain-based desserts (6 percent); dairy-based desserts (6 percent); chicken and chicken mixed dishes as well as sausage, franks, bacon, and ribs (6 percent).[55]

What is the recommended limit for SFA? The 2010 Dietary Guidelines for Americans[55] recommend that we limit saturated fat intake to less than 10 percent of total calories, and that we replace these fats with monounsaturated and/or polyunsaturated fatty acids instead. They state that lowering saturated fat intake to about 7 percent of calories can even further reduce the risk of cardiovascular disease. However, others[136] argue that dietary recommendations to restrict SFA in the diet need to be revised to reflect a range of factors such as: (1) the role of lipid peroxidation in promoting atherogenesis (an effect that is actually more pronounced with polyunsaturated fats than on SFA);

(2) potentially carcinogenic preservatives in processed meats (rich in SFA); (3) preparation and cooking methods used for foods that are traditionally classified as saturated fat foods; (4) potentially *positive* health effects from dairy fat and tropical oils (as described above); (5) farming methods for animals (i.e., grass-fed vs. feed-lot); and (6) the hazards of a diet that is low in fat, but high in refined carbohydrates instead. The debate continues.

So what's the bottom line for SFA? Perhaps the best approach for now, until we know more, is to focus on what we should replace SFA with. For 60 years we've been recommending reduced SFA diets, without providing clear advice on what should replace it. If you look at trends over the past decade, SFA intake has reduced, but it's been replaced by carbohydrates, largely refined carbohydrates. A recent meta-analyses[173] of observational studies clearly showed that if you reduce SFA without paying attention to the replacement, you're simply not going to gain any benefit in terms of cardiovascular disease, especially if you replace the fat with low-fat, high-carbohydrate,

> Simply reducing SFA without regard to what is substituted for it probably isn't going to give you any health benefits. The key is to think about what you are replacing your SFA with.

processed foods. Simply reducing SFA without regard to what is substituted for it probably isn't going to give you any health benefits. The key is to think about what you are replacing your saturated fat with. If our plan is to reduce SFA, then our goal should be to replace dietary SFA fats with healthy fats (poly- and mono-unsaturated fats) so as to get the potential heart-protective benefits of a low-saturated-fat diet.

How To Lower Saturated Fat Intake:

- when preparing foods at home, replace solid fats (e.g., butter and lard) with vegetable oils

- use lower fat cheeses

- purchase fat-free or low-fat milk (**NOTE:** the American Academy of Pediatrics recommends that low-fat/reduced-fat milk not be started before two years of age, but after age two, children should transition to lower fat dairy products);

see discussion regarding consumption of cow's milk *(page 158)*

• trim fat from meat before cooking and eating

Trans Fatty Acids

Although some *trans* fat occurs naturally in foods (i.e., "ruminant" *trans* fatty acids in meat and milk products), most *trans* fats are made during food processing through partial hydrogenation of unsaturated fats *(see Figure 9, page 136)*. These trans fats are referred to as "industrial" or "synthetic" trans fats, and are used primarily to help foods stay fresh longer (i.e., improve shelf life). Trans fats are not essential and provide no known benefit to human health.

Health concerns. Trans fats are thought to pose double trouble for your heart. Research studies show that synthetic trans fat can raise your unhealthy ("bad") LDL cholesterol and lower your healthy ("good") HDL cholesterol, a double whammy that can increase your risk of cardiovascular disease. Trans fats have also been shown to lower LDL particle size (a risk factor for heart disease) and to raise apoB to apoA-I levels, triglycerides (TGs), and Lp(a) levels.[174] Moreover, trans fatty acids have been shown to promote increased body fat and insulin resistance, as well as a state of systemic inflammation in the body.[175-176] A study has even linked consumption of trans fatty acids to a significantly higher risk for depression.[177] This is thought to be mediated by trans fatty acids' affect on increasing proinflammatory cytokines and promoting endothelial dysfunction.[177]

Major sources. You'll find trans fats in partially hydrogenated vegetable oils; commercial baked goods (crackers, cookies, and cakes); commercially fried foods (like doughnuts and French fries); shortening; and some margarines, particularly those that are in stick form. However, in recent years, manufacturers have been using fewer trans fats in foods because of the associated health concerns and consumer awareness of these effects.

What is the limit? The American Heart Association has recommended that no more than one percent of total daily calories be trans fat. So if you consume

2,000 calories, that would be 20 calories, or about 2 grams of trans fat or less per day. The 2010 Dietary Guidelines for Americans[55] are less specific; they simply state that Americans should keep their intake of trans fatty acids as low as possible.

How to Reduce Trans Fat Intake

- Read nutrition labels. Be aware that, in the United States, if a food has less than 0.5 grams of trans fat per serving, the food label can read 0 grams trans fat. Though that's a small amount of trans fat, if you eat multiple servings of foods with less than 0.5 grams of trans fat, you could actually end up taking in quite a bit.

- Look at ingredient lists. The word "shortening" is a clue that the product contains trans fats. If it lists "partially hydrogenated" vegetable oil, it means that it contains at least some trans fat. The terms "fully" or "completely" hydrogenated oil mean that it does *not* contain trans fat, but instead contains saturated fat. Unlike partially hydrogenated oil, the process used to make fully or completely hydrogenated oil does not result in trans-fatty acids. If, on the other hand, the label simply lists "hydrogenated" vegetable oil, it could contain some trans fat.

• Be aware that, although trans fat is showing up less on grocery shelves, some restaurants continue to use it for frying. A large serving of French fries, for example, could contain 5 grams or more of trans fat. Don't be afraid to ask what type of fat goes into their deep fryers.

Solid Fats In General

Solid fats are those with a high percentage of saturated and/or trans fatty acids that are solid at room temperature. Because America is experiencing an ever-expanding obesity epidemic, it is important to watch the amount of discretionary (or nonessential) calories we consume. Discretionary calories consist of "added sugars" and solid fats. Although the 2010 Dietary Guidelines for Americans[55] recommend that we limit our intake of both solid fats and added sugars to no more than 5 to 15 percent of total calories, it is estimated that they actually constitute about 35 percent of calories, on average, or at least 800 calories per day, without contributing to the nutritional adequacy of the diet because they contain no essential nutrients or fiber. Moreover, as the amount of solid fats and/or added sugars increases in the diet, it becomes more difficult to also eat foods with sufficient dietary fiber and essential vitamins and minerals and stay within calorie limits. See *Figure 7 (page 77)* for examples of how much solid fat calories various food products can contain.

Common solid fats. *Common solid fats* include butter, beef fat (tallow, suet), chicken fat, pork fat (lard), stick margarine, and shortening. The fat in liquid milk also is considered to be solid. The saturated and trans fatty acids that are components or ingredients of foods (e.g., shortening in a cake or hydrogenated oils in fried foods) are also considered solid fats.

Major food sources. Major food sources of solid fats in the American diet (as a percentage of total intake) are: grain-based desserts, such as cakes and cookies (11 percent of all solid fat intake); pizza (9 percent); regular (full-fat) cheese (8 percent); sausage, franks, bacon, and ribs (7 percent); and fried white potatoes

(5 percent).[55] Reducing the consumption of solid fats allows for increased intake of nutrient-dense foods without exceeding overall calorie needs.

How to Reduce Solid Fats:

- Eat fewer foods that contain solid fats. This would include: cakes, cookies, and other desserts (that are made with butter, margarine, or shortening); pizza; full-fat cheese; processed and fatty meats (e.g., sausages, hot dogs, bacon, ribs); and ice cream.

- Select lean meats and poultry.

- Choose fat-free or low-fat milk and milk products.

- When cooking, replace solid fats such as butter, beef fat, chicken fat, lard, stick margarine, and shortening with oils, or choose cooking methods that do not add fat.

- Choose baked, steamed, or broiled rather than fried foods.

- Check the Nutrition Facts label and choose foods with little or no saturated fat and no trans fat.

- Limit foods containing partially hydrogenated oils, a major source of trans fats.

FATS TO FAVOR

Monounsaturated Fatty Acids (MUFAs)

Monounsaturated fatty acids (omega-9 fatty acids) have one double bond *(see **Figure 9,** page 136)*. Rich sources include olive oil, peanut oil, canola oil, avocados, nuts, and seeds. Consumption of dietary MUFAs has been shown to promote healthy blood lipids (especially to increase HDL-cholesterol and reduce triglycerides), reduce blood pressure, improve insulin sensitivity, and regulate glucose levels.[178,179] Moreover, provocative new data suggests that MUFAs may be a preferred fuel source for the body, such that that their consumption might favorably influence body composition and ameliorate the risk of obesity.[178] The Academy of Nutrition and Dietetics promotes consuming less than 25 percent of daily calories as MUFA, while the American Heart Association sets a limit of 20 percent MUFA in their guidelines.

MUFAs are a central component of the Mediterranean diet, primarily because of the high consumption of nuts and, particularly, olive oil. Virgin and, especially, extra-virgin olive oil (EVOO) is rich in at least 30 phenolic compounds (such as oleuropein, oleocanthal, tyrosol, and hydroxytyrosol), that other vegetable oils don't have. These compounds are important because they have strong antioxidant, free-radical scavenging, and anti-inflammatory activity.[180] Hydroxytyrosol, in particular, has been known to induce apoptosis (programmed cell death) and cell-cycle arrest in cancer cells. Some research suggests that hydroxytyrosol can also prevent CVD by reducing the expression of adhesion molecules on endothelial cells and preventing the oxidation of LDL particles (both of which contribute to the process of atherosclerosis).[181]

Besides olive oil and nuts, however, Mediterranean diet is also rich in fruits and vegetables, legumes, high-fiber grains, fatty fish, and moderate amounts of red wine—factors that should be taken into consideration. Interestingly, while the Mediterranean diet is a fairly high-fat diet, it has actually been shown to be more effective for weight-loss than a traditional low-fat diet.[182] At the same time, it offers numerous *additional* health benefits, such as improved insulin sensitivity and glycemic control, improved blood pressure, and reduced inflammation, all of which are important in reducing the risk of chronic diseases such as cardiovascular disease, diabetes, and cancer.[183,184] There is even research suggesting that the Mediterranean diet might reduce the risk of depression.[185] If so, people following this type of diet may be less likely to choose poor quality foods (with added sugar and solid fats) in an attempt to obtain temporary escape or relief from their state of distress. This could be an indirect way in which the Mediterranean diet helps with weight control.

Polyunsaturated Fats (PUFAs)

Polyunsaturated fats (PUFAs) are fatty acids that have two or more double bonds *(see **Figure 9**, page 136).* Since the 1960s, the standard nutritional advice has been to substitute vegetable oils, rich in polyunsaturated fatty acids (PUFAs), in place of animal foods rich in SFA. However, at the time this advice first originated, PUFAs were regarded as *one* uniform molecular category. We now know that they are not. There are different types of PUFAs with unique biochemical properties and perhaps divergent clinical, cardiovascular, and other effects. PUFAs can be subdivided into two broad categories. There are the *omega-6* fatty acids (e.g., from corn, safflower, sunflower, cottonseed, and soy oils), and *omega-3* fatty acids (e.g., from fatty fish, flax seed, and walnuts). Two PUFAs, linoleic acid (an omega-6 fatty acid) and alpha-linolenic acid (an omega-3 fatty acid), are considered *essential* to human health because they cannot be manufactured by the body. However, essential fatty acid (EFA) deficiency is quite rare, occurring most often in infants fed EFA-deficient diets.

> There are different types of PUFAs with unique biochemical properties and perhaps divergent clinical cardiovascular, and other effects.

While the evidence for clinical benefits associated with higher intakes of omega-3 PUFAs is well established *(see **Omega-3 Fatty Acids**, page 175)* the effects of the biochemically distinct omega-6 PUFAS remain controversial.

Omega-6 Fatty Acids

In the Sydney Diet Heart Study, a single blinded, randomized controlled trial, it was shown that substituting omega-6 (particularly linoleic acid) in place of SFA actually *increased* the risks of death from all causes, coronary heart disease, and CVD.[186] Why might this be? Although omega-6 PUFAs have indeed been shown to lower LDL cholesterol levels, higher consumption of the omega-6 PUFA linoleic acid has been shown to *increase* the production of oxidized linoleic acid metabolites (OXLAMs), which have been linked mechanistically to the progression of atherosclerosis and increased cardiovascular mortality.[187] This effect is likely to be even stronger under conditions of free radical-mediated oxidative stress produced by cigarette smoking and long-term alcohol exposure. Moreover, higher consumption of omega-6 PUFAs are associated with increased levels of inflammation in the body, as well as a higher carcinogenic potential.

The reality is that omega-6 PUFAs are very bioactive compounds. They are precursors for several different families of bioactive mediators. Some appear, at least in animal models, to regulate all sorts of states, from hunger and addictive behaviors to chronic pain and others.[187] Unfortunately, our understanding of these diverse compounds is still in its infancy. One thing we do know for certain is that if you eat a diet composed of foods raised naturally—whether plant-based or animal-based—as everybody would have done up until about 100 years ago, you'd probably consume a rather small amount of omega-6 PUFAs (about 2 to 3 percent of total calories). The problem today is that most of the vegetable oils that are currently added to packaged and processed foods, at least in the United States, are very high in linoleic acid. And this could prove to be problematic. Certainly these findings challenge worldwide dietary advice to substitute omega-6, or PUFAs in general, for SFA.

> The problem today is that most of the vegetable oils that are currently added to packaged and processed foods, at least in the United States, are very high in linoleic acid, an omega-6 PUFA.

Omega-3 Fatty Acids

The term "omega-3" simply means that the fatty acid has a double bond located at a specific position in the carbon-carbon chain: three carbon atoms from the methyl end. There are three major types of omega-3 fatty acids that are ingested in foods and used by the body: eicosapentaenoic acid (EPA); docosahexanoic acid (DHA); and alpha-linolenic acid (ALA).

EPA and DHA are found naturally in cold-water fish, such as mackerel, tuna, salmon, sturgeon, mullet, bluefish, anchovy, sardines, herring, trout, and menhaden. These fish provide about 1 gram of omega-3 fatty acids in about 3.5 ounces of fish. However, many consumers may have difficulty distinguishing among several health messages about fish consumption. On one hand, we hear of the many health benefits of fish, yet there are warnings about high levels of environmental contaminants with some types of fish.[188] Current FDA warnings apply only to specific groups of individuals: women who may become pregnant or are already pregnant; nursing mothers; and young children. The FDA recommends that people in these categories *avoid* eating shark, swordfish, king mackerel, and tilefish because they contain high levels of mercury.[189] The good news is that five of the most commonly eaten varieties of fish (shrimp, canned light tuna, salmon, pollack, and catfish) are actually quite low in mercury.

ALA is found in *plant* foods such as flaxseed, walnuts, soybeans, chia, pumpkin seeds, and their oils. For more details on food sources and quantities of EPA/DHA/ALA, as well as the issue of safety of fish, see *http://circ.ahajournals.org/content/106/21/2747.full*[190]

Omega-3 fatty acids and heart disease. Interest in omega-3s spiked in the 1970s when scientists observed that the Inuit people of Greenland ate lots of fatty fish and had extremely low rates of heart disease. Since then, it has been established that omega-3 fatty acids reduce the state of inflammation in the body and lower blood triglyceride levels (an independent risk factor for CVD). Interestingly, a 2011 study[191] suggested that a high intake of EPA and DHA may actually protect against some of the detrimental effects commonly associated with obesity. In this study, blood levels of EPA and DHA were taken from Yup'ik Eskimos living in Alaska. Approximately 70 percent of this population is overweight or obese (similar to the rest of the United States), but they consume, on average, 20 times more omega-3 fatty acids from fish than the rest of us. The data showed that those overweight and obese Yup'ik Eskimos who had *lower* blood levels of EPA/DHA were significantly more likely to have both high blood triglycerides and high C-reactive protein (a marker of inflammation), compared to those who had *higher* EPA/DHA levels in their blood. This suggests that omega-3 fatty acids can minimize some of the adverse metabolic factors we typically see in obese individuals. Omega-3 fatty acids have also been shown to avert abnormal heart rhythm and to slow the development of blood clots.

Table 6 lists the American Heart Association (AHA) recommendations for omega-3 fatty acid intake for three different groups of individuals.[192] For those who do *not* have coronary heart disease, the AHA recommends a variety of preferably oily fish at least twice a week (equivalent to about 12 ounces

Table 6. AHA Omega-3 recommendations

Population	AHA Recommendation
Patients without CHD	Eat a variety of (preferably oily) fish at least twice a week. Include oils and foods, rich in linolenic acid (flaxseed, canola, and soybean oils; flaxseed and walnuts)
Patients with documented CHD	Consume 1 gram of EPA+DHA per day, preferably from oily fish. EPA+DHA supplements could be considered in consultation with the physician
Patients needing triglyceride lowering	2–4 grams of EPA+DHA per day provided as capsules under a physician's care

per week). Keep in mind that commercially-fried fish products (e.g., fast food fish) are relatively low in omega-3 fatty acids and high in trans fatty acids (if partially hydrogenated fat is used in preparation). Thus, they do not provide the same benefits as other sources of fish.[192] The guidelines also recommends oils and foods rich in alpha-linolenic acid (ALA), the *plant* form of omega-3s, such as flaxseed and walnuts. However, in order to play a role in the many vital metabolic processes in the body and the brain dietary ALAs must be first converted to DHA and EPA *(see Omega-3 Fatty Acids subsections: "mental health" page 182, "cognitive health" page 184).*

And, unfortunately, the conversion of ALA to EPA is limited, and the conversion to DHA is even more restricted.[193] Thus, ALA ends up being a far less *efficient* source of useable omega-3 fatty acids than EPA or DHA.

Although the AHA does recommend fish oil supplements for certain patients *(Table 6)*, some experts are now questioning their value. In a recent study, published in the *New England Journal of Medicine*,[194] patients with multiple cardiovascular risk factors were given one gram of fish oil per day versus placebo, and the fish oil showed no benefit in terms of CVD reduction. In addition, a few recent meta-analyses[195,196] examining multiple randomized trials, as a whole, have produced rather disappointing results. However, it is important to note that all of the trials examined were *secondary*-prevention, randomized trials, conducted in very high-risk populations (those with multiple risk factors, or a history of CVD), including many subjects who were already taking multiple heart medications (e.g., statins, aspirin, ACE inhibitors), which may very well obscure the effect of omega-3 supplements. So, while *observational epidemiologic* studies *have* shown benefit of omega-3 fatty acids in preventing heart disease (i.e., primary prevention), these randomized controlled trials have not shown benefit in terms of *secondary* prevention (i.e., preventing events in those who already have evidence of the disease process, or preventing recurrent events in those who have already had a cardiac event). What we need are large, *primary* intervention trials in healthy individuals to determine whether omega-3 fatty acids in fish or supplements do indeed prevent cardiovascular events. There is such a trial underway at Brigham and Women's Hospital called VITAL, the vitamin D and OmegA-3 Trial (VITAL).[197] VITAL is a randomized clinical trial in 20,000 U.S. men and women. It is investigating whether taking daily dietary supplements of vitamin D3 (2000 IU) or omega-3 fatty acids (Omacor® fish oil, 1 gram) reduces the risk of developing cancer, heart disease, and stroke in people who do not have a prior history of these illnesses. It will also be looking at other outcomes such as depression, autoimmune disease, diabetes, eye disease, and cognitive decline.

The estimated completion date is summer of 2016. So we will learn more in time.

So, what do we tell our patients in the meantime? Certainly, the randomized trials on fish oil supplements (mentioned above) do not cast doubt on our recommendation to consume at least two servings of dietary fish per week. That is a recommendation from the American Heart Association and many other professional societies, and many studies do suggest benefit. Some of the benefit could be because dietary fish is replacing *other* foods that could increase disease risk, such as red meat or foods high in saturated fat. Thus, we certainly want to continue to recommend at least two servings of fish per week, particularly darker fatty fish, such as salmon and mackerel. It's also important to note that, for those patients who are candidates for prescription omega-3 fatty acid supplements, such as those who have very high triglyceride levels, these meta-analyses findings do not cast doubt on that indication for use. That would still be an appropriate use. And for those patients who are taking fish oil and are doing very well on it, and feel strongly that the fish oil is helping their symptoms or are a benefit to them, there is no strong basis from these studies to recommending that they stop. Fortunately, these studies showed no major risks were associated with fish oil supplements. *(See Omega-3 Fatty Acids subsection, page 188)*

Omega-3 fatty acids and mental health. Omega-3 fatty acids have been shown to play a crucial role in normal brain function. People who do not get enough omega-3 fatty acids in their diets, or who do not maintain a healthy ratio of omega-6 to omega-3 fatty acids *(see Omega-3 Fatty Acids subsection, page 191),* may be at an increased risk for depression,[198] as well as mood and behavioral disorders.[199] This makes sense when one considers that the brain has a high requirement for omega-3 fatty acids, especially DHA. DHA is an important component of nerve cell membranes. It helps nerve cells communicate with each other, which is an essential step in maintaining good mental health. Some,[200-202] but not all, studies[203-206] suggest that the supplementation of omega-3s hold promise as a primary or adjunctive therapy for several neuropsychiatric disorders such as mood disorders, schizophrenia and attention deficit hyperactivity. Mechanistic studies are discovering that omega-3s modulate the fluidity of neuronal membranes. They also have been shown to enhance monoamine transmission (e.g., serotonin and dopamine). Other possible mechanisms included: altering activity of protein kinases and phosphatidylinositol-associated second messenger systems; altering gene expression; and decreasing oxidative stress and inflammation.

The American Psychiatric Association's (APA) Committee on Research on Psychiatric Treatments[207] has concluded that, "the preponderance of epidemiologic and tissue compositional studies supports a protective effect of omega-3 fatty acids, particularly DHA and EPA, in mood disorders." They state that there is a statistically significant benefit for unipolar and bipolar depression, some potential benefit in major depressive disorder and bipolar disorder, but less evidence of benefit in schizophrenia. The APA has provided general guiding principles for the use of omega-3 fatty acids for the treatment of mood disorders, including:

- all adults should eat fatty fish at least two times per week

- patients with mood, impulse control, or psychotic disorders should consume 1 gram daily of EPA + DHA

- a supplement may be useful in patients with mood disorders (1-9 grams daily); use of more than 3 grams daily should be monitored by a physician

The APA guidelines emphasize that these recommendations are *not* intended as a *substitute* for standard treatments for psychiatric disorders, but as a *complement* to these.

Omega-3 fatty acids and cognitive health. Omega-3-fatty acids, EPA/DHA in particular, have a reputation as a "brain food." Let's look at their potential importance at different stages of the lifespan:

- **Early life.** It appears that EPA/DHA have the *greatest* impact when acquired during prenatal and postnatal brain development. According to the World Association of Perinatal Medicine, the Early Nutrition Academy, and the Child Health Foundation, pregnant and lactating women should aim to achieve an average intake of at least 200 mg DHA per day. For healthy term infants, they recommend and fully endorse breastfeeding (which supplies preformed omega-3 fatty acids), as the preferred method of feeding. When breastfeeding is not possible, they recommend use of an infant formula providing DHA at levels 0.2 to 0.5 weight percent of total fat. Dietary omega-3 fatty acids should continue to be supplied after the first six months of life, but currently there is insufficient information to make quantitative recommendations.[208]

- **Childhood.** In a recent study, lower blood levels of omega-3 fatty acids, particularly DHA, in children was linked to poorer reading ability, often a predictor of continued academic achievement, as well as poorer memory and more symptoms of attention-deficit/hyperactivity disorder in the children, even after controlling for sex and socioeconomic status.[209]

- **Young adults.** In a recent study, young adults, ages 18 to 25 years, were supplemented with omega-3 fatty acids (2 g/day of EPA/DHA) for a six-month period.[210] The investigators found that working memory (essential for adaptive reasoning and problem solving) improved dramatically, prompting the project investigator, Bita Moghaddam, Ph.D., professor of neuroscience at the University of Pittsburgh, to comment:

  > Before seeing this data, I would have said it was impossible to move young healthy individuals above their cognitive best…but we found that members of this population can enhance their working memory performance even further, despite already being at the top of their cognitive game.

- **Older adults.** There is great hope that omega-3 fatty acids could be used later in life to improve cognitive function and minimize cognitive decline. Their potential benefit in cognition and dementia include:[100]

1. reduction in CVD and stroke

2. reduction in the synthesis of pro-inflammatory cytokines implicated in the pathogenesis of AD

3. maintenance of brain cell membrane integrity and neuronal function and

4. reduction of beta-amyloid plaque (a prime suspect for AD) by decreasing production and increasing its clearance

While observational and epidemiological studies positively support the use of omega-3 fatty acids (from food and supplements) to preserve cognitive function, unfortunately, results from randomized controlled trials thus far have been short-term, and the results have been inconsistent. One explanation for the inconsistencies could be a timing issue. Perhaps consumers could reap the greatest benefit from DHA supplementation if it is taken well *before* significant cognitive decline has occurred and/or AD has advanced. It could also indicate that a longer follow-up time may be needed to see benefit.[211] However, it's not always that clear-cut.

For example, a meta-analysis of 10 randomized controlled trials in persons with normal cognitive function, mild cognitive impairment, and AD suggested a benefit of omega-3 fatty acids within specific cognitive domains (attention and processing speed) in cognitively impaired individuals without dementia, but found no benefits in healthy subjects or in those with AD.[212] Again, research simply is not always consistent!

Even if no *direct* benefit is observed in clinical trials, use of omega-3 rich foods or supplements could be advised because observational epidemiologic studies have demonstrated their benefit in reducing the risk of cardiovascular events (primary prevention). And, a reduction in cardiovascular risk may, ultimately, lead to improved cognitive outcomes because, it is thought, what is good for the heart is probably also good for the brain.

Omega-3 fatty acid supplements: Are they safe? Of course, an important question, if you are considering supplements, is: Are they safe? As you can see from ***Table 6*** *(page 178)*, if you're trying to lower your blood triglycerides, you'd probably have to have at least two grams per day, generally more in the range of three to four grams per day, to achieve a clinically *significant* reduction in triglycerides.[190] It would be very difficult to achieve this level through diet alone. And, even if you are trying to aim for ~1 gram of omega-3 fatty acids per day to prevent heart disease, improve mood, or enhance cognition, it could be a bit challenging to achieve that with diet, unless you're a person who really enjoys your two-plus servings of fish per week. So for some, supplements may be a good option.

The most commonly reported adverse effects of fish oil are gastrointestinal (GI) upset and a fishy aftertaste. Although not dangerous, the GI upset could be minimized by purchasing enteric coated products, and the bad taste might be avoided by chilling the supplements in the freezer before taking them. The AHA recommends that fish oil supplements be taken "in consultation with a physician," in part because of fish oil's antithrombotic effects. Susceptible individuals, (especially older adults) may run the risk of excessive bleeding (and possibly hemorrhagic stroke) if the supplements are taken in high amounts. If you take blood thinners, anti-platelet drugs, or anti-inflammatory painkillers (like Advil® or Motrin®), talk to your healthcare provider about using omega-3 fatty acids. The combination may increase the risk of bleeding. The same risks could apply to people taking supplements like vitamin E and ginkgo biloba. However, a recent systematic review of the literature, examining 994 older adults, 60 years of age or older, taking doses of EPA and/or DHA ranging from 0.03 grams to 1.86 grams for a period of 6 to 52 weeks, determined that the potential for adverse events appear to be mild to moderate at worst, and are unlikely to be of clinical significance.[213] The NIH states that omega-3 fatty acids are likely safe for most people when taken in low doses (three grams or less per day). For more safety information, see *http://www. nlm.nih.gov/medlineplus/druginfo/natural/993.html.*

When buying a fish oil supplement, be sure to buy one made by an established company who can certify that their products are free of heavy metals such as mercury, lead, and cadmium.[190] The FDA has approved a prescription form of omega-3 fatty acids called Lovaza®, which can deliver higher doses of EPA and DHA than those found in an over-the-counter supplement.

What is the appropriate ratio of omega-6 to omega-3? Several sources indicate that human beings evolved on a diet with a one to one ratio of omega-6 to omega-3 fatty acids, whereas the Western diet today has a ratio closer to 15 to 1 or higher,[214] with some estimates as much as 30 times higher in omega-6.[215] A major reason for this trend is the marked shift in industrialized nations towards higher consumption of omega-6 fatty acids, primarily due to higher intake of vegetable oils rich in linoleic acid (such as corn, sunflower, and safflower oils) in our processed foods. This is a concern because this imbalance has been hypothesized to be a significant risk factor for the rising rate of inflammatory disorders in the United States.[215] Many experts also contend that a high omega-6 to omega-3 ratio is at least partially responsible for the epidemic of autoimmune and cardiovascular diseases that we face today, whereas a higher intake of omega-3 fatty acids (or a lower omega-6 to omega-3 ratio) is protective.[214] While opinions do vary, some experts recommend that a healthy diet contain no more than two to four times more omega-6 fatty acids than omega-3 fatty acids. While there has been much oversimplification regarding the importance of omega-6 to omega-3 PUFA ratio, the reality is that it is very complex because these categories represent different compounds, with differing biochemical effects. The good news is that we can go a long way to improve our omega-6 to omega-3 ratio if we simply reduce our consumption of processed/refined packaged foods— the major source of omega-6 fatty acids in our diet— and work to incorporate more omega-3 fatty acids in the form of fish oil and plant foods rich in omega-3 fatty acids.

Another option to improve the omega-6 to omega-3 ratio, if you are a meat eater, is to choose products derived from grass-fed animals (i.e., free-range) instead of grain-fed. Prior to the 1940s, most beef came from cattle raised on grass. The 1950s gave birth to the feedlot, where farmers began to feed cattle high energy grains to increase efficiency

> We can go a long way to improve our omega-6 to omega-3 ratio if we simply reduce our consumption of processed and packaged foods.

(i.e., fatten up the animals quickly) and to improve marbling. Consumers were initially quite pleased with the change, as they preferred the flavor and overall palatability of meat from grain-fed cattle.[216] However, as new research has begun to reveal significant differences in the fatty acid composition and overall antioxidant content of grass versus grain-fed animals, there has been a shift in consumer demand. Research shows that grass-fed beef not only has a lower overall fat content, but it also has a more favorable omega-6 to omega-3 ratio. It also has a more desirable SFA profile (with more C18:0 cholesterol neutral SFA, and less C14:0 & C16:0 cholesterol elevating SFA) as compared to grain-fed beef.[216] Moreover, grass-fed beef is higher in precursors for vitamin A and E, as well as cancer-fighting antioxidants, compared to grain-fed counterparts. The only downside, from the consumer's perspective, might be the cost and the taste. Because of these differences in fatty acid content, grass-fed beef has a distinct grass flavor and unique cooking qualities that might pose an issue for some when making the transition from grain-fed beef.

Fats for Cooking

I often hear comments and questions such as, "We shouldn't cook with that fat, should we?" It creates free radicals when you heat it, doesn't it?" The whole issue of what constitutes healthy cooking oil is very confusing. And there's lots of misinformation out there, especially floating around on the internet. So let's start with the basics.

Earlier, we divided fats into three broad categories: saturated (SFA); monounsaturated (MUFA); and polyunsaturated (PUFA). As a rule, because they contain more double bonds, PUFA are more easily damaged (or oxidized) by oxygen and heat. Thus, they have a greater tendency to form higher amounts of toxic lipid peroxides, such as 4-hydroxy-2-alkenals, than do SFA or MUFA. However, it's important to know that, while these secondary lipid oxidation products are considered toxic, no upper limit (corresponding to a safe dose) for these compounds has yet been established. Unfortunately, little is known about what dose may constitute a health hazard for humans,[217] though we do know that the body has some natural defense mechanisms against such substances. Some experts have linked exposure to the breakdown products of heated oils to conditions such as atherosclerosis, the forerunner to cardiovascular disease; inflammatory joint disease, including rheumatoid arthritis; pathogenic conditions of the digestive tract; mutagenicity and genotoxicity, properties that often signal carcinogenesis; and teratogenicity, the property of chemicals that leads to the development of birth defects.[218]

PUFAs are considered "damaged" if, at any stage in their manufacture, transport, handling, or use, the oil has been exposed to excessive air, light, or heat. For this reason, oils high in PUFAs should be kept in air-tight/oxygen-free containers and in a cool, dark space. The same goes for nuts or seeds with a high PUFA content, although they are slightly more self-protected than naked oils.

While the type of oil is important, research suggests that there are additional variables that can impact oxidation of oils. For example, the type of food that the oil is contained in may affect the degree of lipid oxidation and degradation because of factors such as the content of transition metals (e.g., iron, copper) and water.[217]

Which oils are best to cook with? Heating an oil changes its characteristics. Oils that are healthy at room temperature may become less healthy when heated above certain temperatures. The best oils to *cook* with are the ones lowest in PUFA. Ideally, choose oils that have a PUFA content of 10 percent or less for cooking. Examples of oils with PUFA contents below 10 percent include olive oil, avocado oil, macadamia oil, palm oil, coconut oil, palm and palm kernel oil, butter, and ghee.

What oils should we avoid heating? Some (not all) experts recommend that we avoid heating oils that have a PUFA content exceeding 20 percent. Examples of oils with PUFA contents exceeding 20 percent include soy, perilla, safflower, sunflower, corn, walnut oil, rice bran oil, and/or peanut oil.

Oils rich in PUFAs have a greater tendency to form toxic lipid peroxides. Thus, it's best to cook with oils that are lower in PUFAS (less than 20 percent), and to store these oils in an airtight container and in cool, dark place.

Proper storage of oils. Remember, oils aren't like fine wine; they don't improve with age. Instead, oils oxidize with age. The process is further accelerated when they are heated and exposed to light. This is especially the case for oils that are high in PUFAs, so keep them in a cool, dark place. The fridge is ideal. Don't be concerned if some of your oils become cloudy or solidified when refrigerated. That's perfectly normal. It doesn't affect their quality. Just place them at room temperature for a few minutes when you want to use them, and they will go back to normal again.

What is the smoke point? The smoke point is simply defined as the temperature at which an oil begins to smoke. The concern is that if you heat oils beyond their smoke points, it could generate toxic fumes and harmful free radicals. It's never a good idea to heat an oil beyond its smoke point. When choosing a cooking oil, its best to match the oil's heat tolerance with the cooking method. But if you try to locate tables of *exact* smoke-point temperatures in cookbooks and food reference books, you will be surprised to see wide variations from chart to chart. Don't believe them. They're really pretty much shots in the dark because there is no such thing as a "typical" olive or peanut oil. Manufacturers of extra-virgin olive oil, for example, have listing their smoke points from just under 200 to well over 400 degrees! But there are some generalities to note. As a rule, vegetable-based oils have higher smoke points than animal-based fats like butter or lard (the main exceptions is hydrogenated vegetable shortening—which you wouldn't want to use anyway because it is a potential source of trans fatty acids. Another factor is the degree of refinement. Refining an oil (i.e., taking out impurities) tends to *increase* the smoke point. It's important to note that any given oil's smoke point does not remain constant over time.

The longer you expose an oil to heat, the lower its smoke point becomes. Thus, fresher oils will have a higher smoke point than the oil you've been cooking with for a while.

Although different sources have printed varying smoke point numbers, the following general categories come from the Cleveland Heart Clinic *(http://health.clevelandclinic.org/2012/05/heart-healthy-cooking-oils-101/)*:

- **High smoke-point oils** are best suited for searing, browning, and deep frying, and include almond, avocado, hazelnut, palm, sunflower, "light" or refined olive oil

- **Medium-to high-smoke point oils** are best suited for baking, oven cooking, or stir frying, and include canola, grape seed, macadamia nut, extra virgin olive , peanut oil

- **Medium smoke-point oils** are best suited for light sautéing, sauces, and low-heat baking, and include corn, hemp, pumpkin seed, sesame, soybean, walnut, and coconut oil

- **No-heat oils** are best suited for dressings, dips, and marinades, and include flaxseed and wheat germ oil

What does it mean when oils are refined? Is that a problem? Some oils are refined to make them more stable and suitable for high temperature cooking. Refining removes most of the flavor and color, but it also raises the smoke point. This makes refined oils perfect for baking and stir-frying. However, the main problem with refined oils is that the refining process also removes many of the nutrients from oils as well. Unrefined oils, by contrast, are simply pressed and bottled, so they retain their original flavor, color, and, most importantly, nutrients. For example, unrefined virgin and extra-virgin olive oil contain a range of phytochemicals, many of which have antioxidant effects (see below).

Which olive oil is the best to buy and use—"light," virgin, or extra virgin (EVOO)? "Light" simply means refined. The advantage of light, in the case of olive oil, is that it would have the highest smoke-point, and therefore be better suited for higher heat cooking. It also tends to be the cheapest form of olive oil.

The disadvantage is that the refining process leaves the oil virtually tasteless and colorless.

At the other end of the quality and price spectrum are the virgin and extra virgin olive oils (EVOO). These are oils that are obtained from the original fruit without being synthetically treated. Once the olives have been picked, washed, and mechanically expressed, no other processing occurs other that the removal of solids by filtration or centrifugation. EVOO is the highest quality and most flavorful olive oil classification, and it has the highest quantity of protective constituents. But, on the other hand, it is also the most expensive, and it has a lower smoke point that refined olive oil. Some chefs might say that they don't want to waste the fine flavor and nutrients of EVOO by cooking it to high temperatures. Instead, they would be more inclined to use it for drizzling, dressings, and dips. So, does it make sense to use your expensive EVOO for cooking? Are the protective polyphenols going to degrade to the point where it no longer has a nutritional advantage over the light or refined olive oil?

Olive oil degradation under heat processing is a complex issue from a chemistry point of view because of the huge amount of different compounds it contains, as well as reactions and interactions taking place under thermal stress. A recent review paper[219] examined the effects of thermal processing of olive oil using different cooking practices, from common frying to boiling and microwave cooking, along with varying operating conditions, such as time, temperature, and food amounts. The study showed that, if we were to compare olive oil to other vegetable oils, under normal cooking conditions with temperatures of up to 350 to 375 degrees Fahrenheit, as is usual for frying and roasting, olive oil's thermal resistance is usually equal or superior to other vegetable oils. This is, in part, a direct consequence of its high MUFA profile. However, even if you compare olive oil to other vegetable oils that have an equivalent amounts of MUFA, olive oil still has better heat stability. This is likely due to the antioxidant capacity of its phenolic compounds, in combination with vitamin E, which provide balanced protection under thermal stress. Still, while olive oil may be more heat stable, thermal stress will undoubtedly modify its chemical profile. Most of its bioactive components, including phenolic compounds and tocopherols (vitamin E) are gradually lost with heating. Therefore, in order to optimize virgin olive oil's profile of health-providing chemical components, its best to reduce heating time to a minimum. When possible, olive oil should be added more closely to the final cooking process. This isn't to say that heating olive oil is harmful; it simply means that after a short heating period, all the *additional* benefit of an expensive high-phytochemical EVOO is lost. From that point forward, most of the advantages of olive oil, especially an EVOO, in comparison with other vegetable oils, are lost, and it behaves primarily as a mixture of mono-unsaturated fatty acids, which is still beneficial from a heart perspective.

So what does all this mean if you're trying to optimize your health while protecting your pocket book? Olive oil is still, in my opinion, the preferred fat. If money is not an issue, buy EVOO and use it for everything, from salad dressing to cooking. If you are watching your wallet and need an oil that you can use regularly in cooking, you can purchase two different olive oils; one EVOO for salad dressing and drizzling, and another, cheaper light olive oil for cooking. Either way, you get the benefit of the MUFAs found in olive oil.

> While all olive oil is actually quite heat resistant as compared to vegetable oils, heat will undoubtedly modify its chemical profile of protective polyphenols. Therefore, it may be best, from an economical perspective, to save your expensive polyphenol-rich extra-virgin olive oil for salad dressings and drizzling, and use cheaper, "light" olive oil for cooking.

TIPS FOR CHOOSING THE HEALTHIEST TYPES OF DIETARY FAT:

- sauté with olive oil; use extra virgin olive oil in salad dressings and marinades

- sprinkle slivered nuts or sunflower seeds on salads instead of bacon bits

- snack on a small handful of nuts rather than potato chips or processed crackers; unsalted peanuts, walnuts, almonds, and pistachios are good choices

- try non-hydrogenated peanut butter or other non-hydrogenated nut-butter spreads on celery, bananas, or whole-grain toast

- add slices of avocado (a MUFA), rather than cheese, to your sandwich

- prepare fish such as salmon and mackerel, instead of meat, twice a week

- consider grass-fed beef to improve the fatty acid profile of the meat

- when choosing an oil for cooking, match the oil's heat tolerance to the cooking method

Chapter 8

Low-Fat vs. Low-Carb:
What Should We Advise Our Patients?

O ver the years, there has been a lot of controversy over what's the best dietary pattern for controlling body weight and improving overall health. Surveys show that grocery shoppers who read nutrition labels look first and foremost at the fat content of foods. The "fat makes you fat" mentality has been seared into our brains. During the 1970s–1990s, the trend was a low-fat diet, not only for weight control, but to promote a healthy heart. But, unfortunately, the problem is that many of those low fat diets of the past 30 to 40 years have actually made us fatter, and appear to have contributed to the epidemic of diabetes we are seeing today! That's primarily because when people try to follow very low-fat diets, in many cases, they end up eating more "low-fat" or "fat-free" *processed* foods added to the marketplace. But, while these products are indeed lower in fat, they also contain a lot more sugar and refined carbohydrates. As a result, paradoxically, a low-fat diet can end up being far less healthy than it would be if they incorporated higher fat foods, such as nuts and seeds. Dr. Atkins and others argued that, because people were gaining weight on the low-fat diets, it must be that the carbs that were to blame, thus heralding in another round of the low-carb craze, demonizing carbs. To make things even more confusing, the Atkins diet contended that SFA could be eaten to the heart's delight—bacon double cheeseburgers for all—so long as carbs were avoided. And, thus, the low-carb, low-fat pendulum continued to swing back and forth. The result? People just got more and more confused. And the barrage of contradictory and confusing information only served to create the core problem: people were simply not eating enough real, whole foods.

We've all learned that the fundamental cause of obesity is an excess of calories. That too much of any calories—whether from protein, fat, or carbohydrates (the energy, or calorie-yielding macronutrients)—will inevitably pack on the pounds. And all of this stems from the first law of thermodynamics, which states that energy can neither be created nor destroyed. So, in other words, energy, or calories, consumed has to either be converted to a useful form (metabolized), excreted, or stored (as in fat tissue). But is there more to the story than just calories?

There are only three calorie-yielding macronutrients (protein, fat, and carbs), and you *do* have to eat (you need calories to survive). So if one of these macronutrients goes down, another *has* to go up. And, because fat is the most dense source of calories (fat has 9 calories per gram, whereas carbs and protein have only 4 calories per gram), you'd think it would be best to limit fat. But, the fact of the matter is that we need at least some fats in order for our bodies to function normally. If you avoid *all* fat, you may be at risk of getting insufficient amounts of essential fatty acids. Fat is also important to help us absorb fat-soluble vitamins and phytochemicals, such as beta carotene. It also gives us a sense of fullness, or satiety. So if you reduce your fat intake too drastically, you may be thinking about food all day, or even end up bingeing, when your resolve to restrict weakens after a long hard, stressful day.

The carb-fat controversy is probably one of the most daunting in all of nutrition. Both camps—the low carb and the low fat—can offer logical rationale to persuade you to join their teams. But the main problem with both sides is their simple, dichotomous approach to nutrition. The reality is that not all carbs are the same, just like not all fat is the same. Some carbs, such as the high-fiber carbs found in whole foods such as fruits, vegetables, beans, and grains, are strikingly different than the carbs you would find in a processed, low-fat food. The main problem with the original low-carb diet is that no distinctions were being made between refined carbs (sugar and white flour, commonly found in processed food) and natural carbohydrates (typically found in plants).

Likewise, not all fats are the same. The hydrogenated soybean oil you find in a processed food product, such a stick margarine, is strikingly different that fats you find in EVOO or nuts. Thus, we do our patients/ clients a great disservice when we clump these macronutrients together in one group, saying that carbs are carbs and fats are fats.

> Not all calories are alike from a metabolic perspective.

While carbs do have 4 calories per gram, how that carb will affect your weight and your metabolic state greatly depends upon its fiber and/or its glycemic load. It is the quality of the carbs that is most important; this is what is going to affect the metabolic consequences of a particular diet. Likewise, while fats have 9 calories per gram, the amount and position(s) of its double bond(s), as well as other constituents in the foods that contain that fat, can have varying effects on a persons' health.

The new mindset is that all the focus on calories has been ill-placed—that we have made a fundamental error in our thinking about obesity. It is not the

Instead of considering obesity to be a disorder of energy balance, we should instead consider it to be more akin to a hormonal defect, an insulin defect—the result of a pancreas attempting to oversecrete insulin in response to a poor quality, refined carbohydrate diet.[220]

energy or calorie content of foods—whether steak, bread, soda, or avocados—that makes them fattening. It is instead the effects of these foods, carbohydrates in particular, on our hormones that determine whether we accumulate fat.[220] If we are consuming a diet high in refined carbohydrates, high glycemic load foods, and we keep cranking out insulin to help with the situation, then, over time, the body becomes more and more resistant to that insulin, and, subsequently, cranks out even *more* insulin in an attempt to compensate. This is a concern because insulin is the key hormone for stimulating fat accumulation in the body. Insulin tells fat cells to store fat. And as long as insulin levels remain high, fat cells stubbornly hang on to that fat. So, indeed, all calories really aren't the same after all. The key is the quality of calories and how it affects hormone balance in the body.

Insulin resistance, driven by lots of added sugars and refined carbs, not only explains why we get fat, but also why rates of diabetes are rising as well.

A recent study[221] of overweight and obese adults examined differences in energy expenditure after being randomized to three different, calorie-equivalent diets: a low-fat diet (LF) diet; a low-glycemic-index diet (LGI); and a very low-carbohydrate (VLC) diet. It found that the LF group had the greatest reduction in energy expenditure (i.e., their metabolism slowed down the most). This diet also produced changes in serum leptin (a hormone made by fat cells that promotes satiety) that would predict weight regain. In contrast, the VLC diet had the most beneficial effects on energy expenditure and several metabolic syndrome components, but this restrictive regimen resulted in increased cortisol levels (a stress hormone) and higher C-reactive protein (a marker of inflammation). However, while the LGI had qualitatively similar, though smaller, metabolic benefits to the VLC diet, it was not associated with the deleterious effects on physiological stress and chronic inflammation. These findings suggest that a strategy to reduce glycemic load, rather than dietary fat or carbohydrates, may be most advantageous for accomplishing both weight loss maintenance and cardiovascular disease prevention. The authors reinforce the message that a low-glycemic index diet is best for weight loss *and* cardiovascular disease prevention, and reinforces the concept that not all calories are alike from a metabolic perspective.

Clearly, the best approach, over the long-term, would be to avoid restriction of any major nutrient—either fat or carbohydrate—and instead focus on the quality of nutrients. This is not to say that the number of calories isn't important; instead, it's saying that if we focus on improving the quality of our calories, work on improving our relationship with food, as well as staying active, reducing stress, and getting sufficient healthy sleep, then we won't have to think so much about calories. Our bodies will take care of themselves if we give them what they need.

Chapter 9

Salt: Should We Pass (Up) the Shaker?

The role of sodium in the body. Sodium is primarily consumed in the diet in the form of salt (a.k.a., sodium chloride), which is about 40 percent sodium. Sodium is essential for normal body function. It helps maintain the right fluid balance in the body, helps transmit nerve impulses, and influences the contraction and relaxation of muscles. However, it is only needed in relatively small quantities, unless substantial sweating occurs. In ancient times, humans probably consumed less than 0.25 grams of salt per day. However, today, virtually *all* Americans consume significantly more sodium than they actually need.

How much sodium does the body need? The Institute of Medicine[222] has set Adequate Intake (AI) levels for sodium based on the amount required to meet the sodium needs of most healthy and moderately active individuals. The AI levels for sodium are as follows:

- **children ages one to three years** – 1,000 mg per day

- **children ages four to eight years** – 1,200 mg per day

- **individuals ages 9 to 50 years** – 1,500 mg per day

- **individuals ages 51 to 70 years** – 1,300 mg per day (their calorie requirements are lower)

- **individuals age 71 years and older** – 1,200 mg per day

Why is sodium (salt) added to foods? Back around 5,000 years ago, it was the Chinese who discovered that salt could be used to preserve food. It helps prevent food from spoiling by inhibiting the growth of bacteria, yeast, and mold. But once refrigerators

> Virtually *all* Americans consume more sodium than they actually need.

and freezers became commonplace, salt was no longer needed for preservation, and intake started to decline.[223] But salt (sodium chloride) serves other purposes besides allowing products to sit on the shelves for months on end. The food industry is hooked on salt because it's viewed, essentially, as a miracle ingredient. It brings out the flavors in foods. It accentuates the sweetness in cakes and cookies (makes sweet taste sweeter). It even enhances the positive sensory attributes of those foods that would otherwise seem unpalatable. For example, salt can mask the "off-notes" in flavors that are inherent to many processed foods, such as the metallic or chemical aftertaste you might find in products, such as soft drinks.[1] It helps foods retain moisture, reducing the perception of dryness in foods such as crackers and pretzels. It can even enhance texture (e.g., adding crunch to foods such as crackers, chips, and frozen waffles). When the food industry discovered that salt can make cheap, unpalatable food edible at virtually no cost, well, it was a no-brainer. From that point on, the intake of salt from processed foods in the Western world began to climb. Moreover, according to some, because salt

> The food industry is hooked on salt because it is viewed as a miracle ingredient. Salt can make cheap unpalatable food edible at virtually no cost.

is a major determinant of thirst, and many of the largest snack firms in the world also have soft-drink components of their companies, they have a vested interest in keeping processed foods salty so as to keep profits coming in.[223]

The hedonic (pleasurable) impact of salt. The ability of food manufacturers to find synergy in the interplay of their key ingredients is not limited to fat and sugar, of course. The true magic comes when they add in the third pillar of processed foods: salt.[1] While most palatable foods contain a combination of sugar, fat, and salt, if they have the right *mix* of these ingredients, they reach the "bliss point" and become hyperpalatable,[3] more stimulating. According to Moss,[1] salt is considered the "magical ingredient" for the food industry because it provides a cheap burst of flavor. Just a pinch of salt will make the flavor explode. Adding lots of salt is the cheapest and easiest way to make products palatable. The power of salt in food is summed up well by the industry's largest supplier of salt, Cargill, which states in its sales literature, "People love salt. Among the basic tastes—sweet, sour, bitter, salty—salt is one of the hardest ones to live without. And it's no wonder. Salt gives food their taste appeal—in everything from bacon, pizza, cheese and French fries to pickles, salad dressings, snacks food and baked goods." But the reality is that people don't just love salt, they *crave* salty foods.

Interestingly, however, it appears that, unlike sugar or sweetness, we're not *born* with a preference for salt. Babies do not like salt. In fact, they don't like it all, at least not until they're about six months old. And, even then, they have to be taught, to be coaxed, to like it. But with time and continued exposure, they start to like it. According to Moss,[1] "With this revelation, the industry's heavy use of salt moves from the realm of merely satisfying America's craving for salt to creating a craving where none exists." Thus, this very early dietary exposure can play a strong influential role in shaping the salty taste preferences of infants and young children. Once they learn to like it, salt can have a deep and lasting effect on their eating habits.[224] The implication here is that if one wants to reduce salt in the population as a whole, then it's important to start early, because infants and children are very vulnerable.

Thus, while we may not be born craving salt, we can certainly become salt cravers. But why the eventual allure? While it certainly makes sense from a survival perspective that our pleasure centers ("Twinkie" circuits) would light up for fat and carbs (sugar) because these macronutrients provide energy/calories important for survival, the question is: what does salt provide? Well, remember that tongue map we talked about earlier? Well, it turns out that, not only was it wrong for sweet flavors, it was wrong for salty flavors too. While the tongue map depicts salt as having a very limited zone, the truth is that we can taste salty foods all through the mouth. And, in fact, the body has receptors for salt extending all the way down to the gut. Such extensive wiring for salt must be there for a reason, right? According to Moss,[1] the desire for salt could have some grounding in evolutionary history. He argues that when everything lived in the ocean, animals had no problem getting the sodium they needed to survive. They wallowed in salty water. However, once on land, where the early climate was hot and dry, the pre-human mouths/guts may have developed the salty taste receptors as a means of ensuring that their owners didn't forget about salt when they foraged for food. Plausible? Perhaps—but that desire for salty food is certainly wreaking havoc on our health today.

Some experts in the field believe that the high amount of salt in processed foods is one of the most important reasons for the current obesity epidemic as it leads to higher consumption of poor quality foods because it makes food more desirable as it aims to achieve the bliss point. The more potent and multisensory the product is, the greater the reward we experience and the greater our drive is to consume *more* of that product.[4] Palatability is clearly the primary driver of food choices. When we get used to the taste of higher sodium foods, it raises our "salt threshold," and other, less salty, foods (such a real, whole foods) often taste bland in comparison.

Problems associated with excess sodium consumption.
It used to be that salt was viewed in a very positive light. We've all heard expressions such as "the salt of the earth." But then, around the late 1980s, a flurry of new reports and scientific studies focused the country's attention on a growing health problem: high blood pressure. A public health survey reported that one in four Americans was afflicted by this conditions, also known as hypertension, a condition often referred to as a "silent killer", because many people didn't even know they had it (and many *still* today don't know that they have it!). And while, at the time, health experts weren't exactly sure what was causing it, the top factors on the list were obesity, smoking, and salt. So, from that point on, salt became targeted as more of a villain. And while a little bit of sodium is essential, the problem was that Americans were consuming way too much—as much as 10 to 20 times—the amount of sodium the body needed, or could handle.

The problem with sodium is that it pulls fluid into the blood, which then raises the blood volume and, ultimately, blood pressure. This forces the heart to pump harder. The result? High blood pressure, a serious health condition that can put us at risk for some of America's biggest killers—cardiovascular disease, heart failure, kidney disease, and stroke.

According to NHANES 2007–2008 data, 28.5 percent of U.S. adults (older than 18 years of age) have hypertension.[225] Of these, 80.7 percent are aware of their condition, 72.5 percent are receiving pharmacologic treatment, and in approximately 50 percent, the hypertension is controlled (a blood pressure reading of lower than 140/90 has been achieved). Roughly one-third of adults currently have *pre*hypertension, the designation used to identify individuals at high risk of developing hypertension, so that preventive measures can be taken. It is important to realize that, even if your blood pressure is currently within the normal range, chances are that it will eventually go up. It has been estimated that individuals who are normotensive at age 55 years have a 90 percent lifetime risk for eventually developing hypertension.[226] Hypertension is of particular concern for women because it contributes to more preventable deaths in women than any other preventable condition.[227] Hypertension is also a major concern for African-Americans, because the prevalence of hypertension among this group is among the highest in the world and continues to increase. But keep in mind that, although the rates of hypertension are higher in certain populations, hypertension is a major problem *across the board*. Rates of high blood pressure have been increasing in the entire population, even in children and adolescents.

> No one is immune to the adverse effects of excess sodium. The benefit of sodium reduction extends to the vast majority of the population, including children and young adults.

A strong body of evidence documents that, in general, as sodium intake increases, so does blood pressure. Thus, while some may have the impression that sodium reduction is only necessary for *certain* individuals (those at high risk of developing hypertension, such as African-

Americans and older adults), the reality is that *no one* is immune to the adverse effects of excess sodium. While certain groups are most likely to benefit from a lower sodium diet, the benefit of sodium reduction extends to the vast majority of the population, including children and young adults.[228]

A study published in *The New England Journal of Medicine* in 2010 used sophisticated, computerized, predictive modeling to estimate the benefit of a population-wide reduction in sodium.[228] It determined that a sodium reduction of 1,200 mg per day would reduce the annual number of new cases of coronary heart disease by 60,000, to 120,000, and number of new cases of stroke by 32,000, to 66,000. The researchers estimated that if Americans halved their sodium intake, as many as 150,000 premature deaths could be prevented each year.

CURRENT RECOMMENDATIONS FOR SODIUM/SALT— CAN YOU BELIEVE IT IS STILL CONTROVERSIAL?

The 2010 Dietary Guidelines for Americans[55] recommend a daily limit of less than 2,300 mg of sodium (or less than 5.8 grams of salt, about one teaspoon) for persons two years of age or older. However, a lower target of less than 1,500 mg of sodium (3.7 grams of salt) per day is recommended for *most* adults (persons over 40 years of age, African-Americans, and persons with hypertension). Similarly, the 2011 American Heart Association guidelines for the prevention of cardiovascular disease in women recommend no more than 1,500 mg of sodium per day.[77]

However, in the spring of 2013, the Institute of Medicine came out with a report entitled: *Sodium Intake in Populations: Assessment of Evidence*[229] that challenged earlier recommendations by the Dietary Guidelines for Americans and the American Heart Association. It stated that, while the body of evidence does show that reducing sodium intake reduces blood pressure and risk of CVD and stroke, the evidence is not strong enough, or consistent enough, to determine whether sodium intakes *specifically below 2,300 mg daily* are actually beneficial. In fact, it raised concern that for some groups, such as patients who

SODIUM RECOMMENDATIONS FROM THE 2010 DIETARY GUIDELINES FOR AMERICANS & THE AMERICAN HEART ASSOCIATION[55]

- *Persons 2 years of age or older:* limit sodium to less than 2,300 mg per day (or about 5.8 grams of salt, about 1 tsp).[55]

- *Persons 51 years of age or older, and individuals of any age who are African-American, or who have hypertension, diabetes, or chronic kidney disease:* limit sodium to 1,500 mg per day (or less than 3.7 grams of salt per day).[55]

- The American Heart Association states that **all women** should limit their sodium intake to 1,500 mg per day.[77]

have a diagnosis of moderate or severe congestive heart failure and are receiving certain aggressive therapeutic treatments, low sodium intakes may actually *increase* health risks. Moreover, it concluded that the data is not strong enough to recommend an *even lower* limit (1,500 mg daily) for certain subgroups (i.e., those 51 years of age and older, African-Americans, and those with hypertension, diabetes or chronic kidney disease). The core problems the committee pointed to were: (1) the lack of standardized methodological approaches for measuring sodium intake, so that we can compare, across different studies, and (2) the need for methods to account for confounding factors in various dietary studies. The committee pointed to the need for more randomized controlled trials, particularly in higher-risk subgroups such as African-Americans and adults 51 years of age and older, so as to strengthen our recommendations. However, it's important to know that, since its release, this report has gotten a lot of criticism. One reason for this is that it claims that we don't have enough quality studies, but it failed to consider a very important, new rigorous trial called the DASH Sodium Trial,[230] which did address some of the methodological issues that have plagued research in this field. This study compared three different levels of sodium: (1) Roughly 1,500 mg daily (the more restrictive recommendation for certain subgroups); (2) 2,300 mg daily (the usual recommendation); and (3) About 3,500 mg daily (equivalent to a typical American diet). Importantly, it was a 16-week feeding study, meaning that every meal was provided to the subjects (410 individuals) for about 16 weeks. Not surprisingly, the study showed a progressive dose-response relationship; the higher the sodium intake, the higher the blood pressure levels. But, importantly, the dose-response relationship was actually *steeper* at levels between 1,500 and 2,300 mg daily, meaning that the greatest drop in blood pressure occurred when subjects restricted sodium to an intake within this range. The study also demonstrated that the results for certain subgroups that are often referred to as "salt sensitive"—African-Americans and older individuals—were the most striking. Thus, while earlier scientific studies may have been plagued by methodological issues, this study shows that, if done well, research can demonstrate the benefits of a lower sodium intake.

How much sodium are we currently consuming? Unfortunately, as shown in *Figure 12* America's sodium consumption far exceeds current public health recommendations. According to a CDC report[231] based on survey data collected from 2005 to 2006, only 9.6 percent of all U.S. adults meet their applicable recommended limit, and, specifically, only 5.5 percent of adults who consumed less than

Figure 12. *Average daily salt intake, 2005-2006*

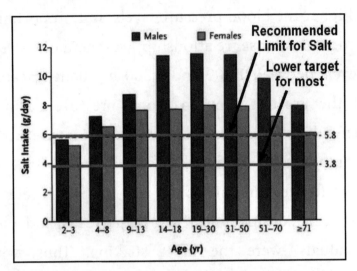

Source: National Cancer Institute, Sources of sodium among the U.S. Population, 2005–2006. Bethesda, MD: National Cancer Institute. http://riskfactor.cancer.gov/diet/foodsources/sodium.

the 1,500 mg daily amount put forth by the Dietary Guidelines for Americans, actually consumed that little. In fact, it is estimated that the average American man consumes about 10.4 grams of salt (or 4,000 mg of sodium) a day, far exceeding the recommended target *(see Figure 12)*.[55,232] And the average woman consumes about 7.3 grams of salt (or about 2,900 mg of sodium) per day.[55,232]

Why is it so difficult to reduce our sodium consumption? In the past four decades, Americans'

Figure 13. *Sources of sodium in U.S. diet*[110]

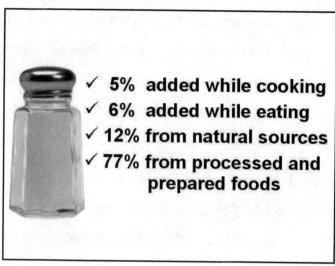

✓ 5% added while cooking
✓ 6% added while eating
✓ 12% from natural sources
✓ 77% from processed and prepared foods

salt consumption has risen dramatically. Reducing sodium is challenging, in part, because, as shown in *Figure 13*, in most developed countries, including the United States, approximately 75 percent to 80 percent of the sodium in the typical U.S. diet comes from foods that are processed and prepared, and not from salt added during food preparation or consumption. In fact, the much-maligned saltshaker only delivers about 6 percent of our sodium intake.[228,233] Thus, simply getting people to stop using "visible" salt is only the tip of the iceberg when it comes to reducing sodium consumption.

That's the main reason why, despite 40 years of health advocates struggling to educate citizens about reducing salt intake, the fact of the matter is that per capita consumption actually appears to be increasing or is, at best, unchanged. But where is the sodium coming from?

- **Natural sources:** this includes all vegetables and dairy products such as milk, meat, and shellfish; however, very little sodium occurs naturally

- **In the kitchen and at the table:** many recipes call for salt; in addition, people often salt their food at the table, or use condiments, such as catsup and soy sauce, that can contain quite a bit of sodium

- **Processed foods:** a major source is breads and cereals (an estimated 33 to 40 percent of our sodium typically comes from this category, in part because they are consumed so frequently); other important sources include prepared dinners such as pasta, meat, and egg dishes; cold cuts and bacon; cheese; soups; and fast foods

It's important to keep in mind that sodium is not just found in the form of salt; food companies are adding dozens of different sodium-based compounds (e.g., sodium citrate, sodium phosphate, and sodium acid pyrophosphate) to processed foods to delay the onset of bacterial decay, bind ingredients, and blend mixtures of foods, among others.

Sodium is so pervasive in the average U.S. diet. We can attempt to put down the salt shaker and cut down on salty snacks, but there's still so much sodium packed into processed foods that trying to reduce it is a real challenge. And it is especially difficult for families with limited incomes who tend to rely more on processed or packed foods and canned fruits and vegetables than they do on fresh foods.

Reducing sodium is challenging, in part because 75 to 80 percent of the salt in the U.S. diet comes from processed foods, not salt added during food preparation or consumption.[228,233]

Some examples of where salt is hiding (total sodium content, in milligrams)*:

- one 8-ounce serving of milk – 130 mg of sodium

- one slice of commercial whole-wheat bread – 148 mg of sodium

- one slice of commercial white bread – 170 mg of sodium

- one cup of Cheerios – 213 mg of sodium

- one cup of Total Raisin Bran – 239 mg of sodium

- one cup of canned sweet corn – 571 mg of sodium

- one slice of fast food pepperoni pizza – 670 mg of sodium

- one fast-food English muffin with cheese and Canadian bacon – 729 mg of sodium

- one fast food fish sandwich with tartar sauce and cheese – 939 mg of sodium

- one fast food chicken fillet sandwich, plain – 959 mg of sodium

- one corndog – 973 mg of sodium

- one single, large patty, cheeseburger with condiments – 1,108 mg of sodium

- one large fast food taco – 1,233 mg of sodium

Source: USDA National Nutrient Database. www.nal.usda.gov/ fnic/foodcomp/Data/SR18/nutrlist/sr18a307.pdf

Thus, clearly, the major reason we are taking in more salt is that we are depending on processed and prepared foods to feed ourselves. And, as a result, we are essentially being "assaulted by salt." According to Moss's research,[1] processed food companies haven't just been adding salt, they've literally been dumping sack after sack into their boxed macaroni and cheese, their canned spaghetti and meatballs, their salad dressings, tomato sauces, pizza and soups. And this has been the case even in the products that are being promoted specifically for people who want to lose weight or manage their diabetes. Even the low-fat, low-sugar versions of their products deliver huge doses of salt. The fact of the matter is: the salting of processed food has become an easy way to increase

> The salting of processed food has become a way to increase sales and encourage consumption.

sales and encourage consumption.

To make matters worse, over time, our taste buds and our bodies have adapted to higher and higher levels of salt, so that we crave way more than we really need to function. And, although people generally know that they should limit their sodium intake, sodium is simply not a "top of mind" nutrition issue for most consumers in the United States. They've gotten accustomed to higher levels of sodium in processed and restaurant foods, and have difficulty adjusting to foods with healthier levels of sodium. But, the good news is that the preference for salty taste can be changed, with time and with patience.[234]

SHOULD THE INDUSTRY BE REGULATED?

For those who have the time and resources to cook meals from scratch, it's pretty easy to reduce sodium consumption. But let's face it—these days, most busy Americans depend on grocery stores (for processed convenience foods) and restaurants for much of their food. This means that consumers have little *direct* control over how much sodium is being added to their food. But the current level of sodium in the food supply—added by food manufacturers, foodservice operators, and restaurants—is simply too high to be considered "safe."[234] In order to really succeed in a population-wide effort to reduce sodium intake, consumers need help. As it stands now, despite 40 years of salt reduction initiatives—focused mainly on consumer education and *voluntary* salt reduction by the food industry—sodium consumption has gone up, not down. So, rather than training 5 billion people to reduce sodium intake by reading food labels, the food industry needs come on board to reduce the amount of sodium that they routinely provide in their products. "Without major change, hypertension and cardiovascular disease rates will continue to rise, and consumers, who have little choice, will pay the price for the food industry's inaction."[234]

We need a food system where making the healthy choice is the *easy* one, not the *hard* one. Given the considerable overconsumption of sodium in this country, and the important effect of sodium on blood pressure and disease, critical policy and environmental changes are required. According to the Institute of Medicine, what is needed is a coordinated effort to reduce sodium in foods *across the board* by manufacturers and restaurants to create a level playing field for the food industry.[234] All segments of the food industry would be adhering to the same reductions and none would be at a disadvantage. The Institute of Medicine recommends that the FDA set *mandatory* national standards for the sodium content in foods—not banning the addition of salt to foods outright, but beginning the process of reducing excess sodium in processed foods and menu items to a safer level.[234] They recommend that the reduction in sodium content of foods be carried out gradually, in a systematic, stepwise process. That way, sodium reduction could be successfully accomplished without affecting consumer enjoyment of food products. The FDA has yet to act on this request. While opponents of this approach may question whether the government ("Big Brother") should be allowed to influence how or what we eat, perhaps a more important question might be: should the food industry be allowed to serve food that makes us sick and kills us?

The good news is that we are making some progress in the right direction. For example, a nationwide coalition, the National Salt Reduction Initiative (NSRI), was initiated by New York City to have discussions with food manufacturers regarding setting voluntary benchmarks for lowering the sodium content of specific food products. As of 2012, 28 packaged food and restaurant companies, many of them large national players such as Kraft, Target, and Subway, have committed to the targets.[235]

RECOMMENDATIONS FOR LOWERING SODIUM INTAKE

1. **Consume more fresh food**, such as fresh fruits, vegetables, lean meats, poultry, fish, and unprocessed grains. These foods are naturally low in sodium. Make sure your fresh meat has not been injected with a sodium-containing solution— look on the label or ask the butcher. Buy plain,

whole-grain rice and pasta instead of white pasta and pasta that has added seasonings.

2. **Prepare more food at home**, instead of eating pre-prepared or restaurant foods. That way you have more control over the amount of sodium you are consuming.

3. **Avoid adding salt to homemade dishes/use alternative seasonings** by trading in your salt shaker for the pepper shaker. Learn to use spices and herbs (e.g. basil, cilantro, curry, ginger, oregano, paprika, rosemary, sage, or turmeric) and lemon to enhance the taste of food as alternatives to salt. Be aware that some salt substitutes, or "light" salts, contain a mixture of table salt and other ingredients. So, depending on how much you use, you could consume too much sodium from such products. In addition, many salt substitutes contain potassium chloride. Although potassium is beneficial *(see "The role of potassium," page 244)*, too much can be harmful if you have kidney problems or are taking certain medications for

Figure 14. Read food labels

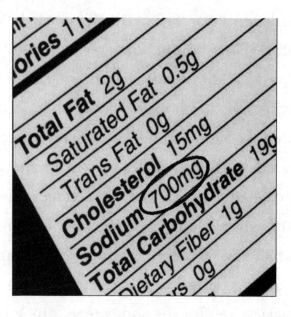

hypertension or congestive heart failure that cause potassium retention.

4. At the table, **taste food before adding salt.**

5. **Limit the use of sodium-laden condiments** such as soy sauce, salad dressings, sauces, dips, catsup, mustard, and relish.

6. When shopping, **read food labels** *(see Figure 14).* Look for lower-sodium varieties of cereals, crackers, chips, pretzels, nuts, pasta sauces, canned

soups, and vegetables, or any foods that might have low-salt options. Select those labeled "reduced sodium," "low sodium," or "no salt added." Choose the brand that is lower in sodium and tastes just as acceptable, or almost as acceptable, as the non-reduced sodium brand. If you're interested in prepared spaghetti sauces, for example, you can get spaghetti sauces that have huge amounts of sodium (over 900 mg per serving), or you can get ones that have about 300 mg per serving, and some have 50 mg per serving. It's important to look by label class (eg., breads and cereals). In general, it's best to limit any product that has over 300 to 400 mg of sodium per serving, because that will give you a big bang for the buck. In terms of cereals, I think you can aim for even less. You could aim for products that have less than 100 mg per serving.

7. **Realize that it may take 8 to 12 weeks for a shift in taste preference to occur.** Granted, a lower sodium variety may not taste that great at first. In fact, some might describe these foods as tasting like "shoe leather" or "cardboard." But stick

with it! There some classic studies from the 1970s in which people gradually reduced their sodium, and within a month or so, the foods that they *used* to like actually tasted too salty. Your taste for salt is acquired, and you can learn to enjoy less. If you decrease your use of salt gradually, your taste sensors will eventually adjust to the lower sodium level. The goal is to get to a point where you go back to some of the saltier foods you *used* to eat, and you realize that you just don't like them anymore because they taste *too* salty! Not only will your preference for salt diminish over time, but you will start to enjoy the taste of the food itself, which was masked by all that salt! The salt-sensitive taste buds in your mouths—the same ones that have grown used to a bombardment of salty foods—will become more sensitive to salt, so you will need less salt to experience its pleasures.

What about sea salt? Sea salt has become the rage lately, with manufacturers boasting their use of it as an alternative to regular table salt. The reality is that sea salt and table salt both contain sodium chloride and have the same basic nutritional value. Sea salt is less processed (it's just evaporated seawater), so it might have a *little more* trace minerals than table salt (which is mined from underground processed sal deposits). And, there is no iodine added to sea salt as there is with table salt. However, when it comes to the sodium content, there's not a lot of difference. Sea salt contains *slightly* less sodium *only* because it is *less fine* than table salt. Therefore, 1 tablespoon of table salt has a little more sodium than 1 tablespoon of sea salt. The larger, more irregular granules of sea salt are said to provide a slightly crunchy and more briny flavor. So the real differences between sea salt and table salt are the taste, texture, and processing, not the chemical makeup. Regardless of which type of salt you prefer, you should aim to keep your sodium consumption below 2,300 mg per day.

The role of potassium. Although reducing sodium is important to control blood pressure, getting sufficient potassium in the diet is just as important. Research shows that a potassium deficit plays a critical role in the development of hypertension and its cardiovascular sequelae.[236] Unfortunately, compared with diets that are based on natural foods, diets based on processed foods are not only **high in sodium**, but also **low in potassium**.[236] This is a concern because human kidneys are designed to *conserve* sodium and *excrete* potassium. This mechanism served pre-historic humans (who consumed a sodium-poor, potassium-rich diet) quite well. Unfortunately, our kidneys have been unable to adapt to our modern sodium-rich, potassium-poor diet. Therefore, it is important to rebalance sodium and potassium intake by following the tips above, as well as by emphasizing high-potassium foods, such as fresh fruits and vegetables, in the diet.

According to recommendations by the CDC and the Institute of Medicine,[234] adults should consume at least 4.7 grams of potassium per day to lower blood pressure, blunt the effects of salt, and reduce the risk of kidney stones and bone loss. It is estimated, however, that most American women age 31 to 50 years consume no more than half of the recommended amount of potassium, and men's intake is only moderately higher.[234] One factor that may motivate people to get more potassium is a recent meta-analysis[237] that showed that a higher potassium intake can cut the risk of stroke by at least 20 percent.

Exercise, sodium sensitivity, and blood pressure. Research suggests that your sensitivity to sodium may very well depend on how active you are.[238] Scientists looked at the blood pressure change in 1,906 Han Chinese adults who participated in the Genetic Epidemiology Network of Salt Sensitivity Study—a large project aimed at identifying genetic and environmental factors that contribute to salt sensitivity. First, they divided the participants into four groups based on their physical activity questionnaires, ranging from "very active" to "quite sedentary." Each group was put on a one-week, low-sodium diet (3,000 mg per day), and then switched to a one-week, high-sodium diet (18,000 mg per day). Meanwhile, scientists analyzed the participants' blood pressure levels to see to what extent their blood pressures rose after changing to a high sodium diet. Interestingly, the results showed that the more physically active the participants were, the *less likely* they were to have increased blood pressure in response to a high-salt diet. On the other hand, the more sedentary they were, the *more likely* they were to have an increase in blood pressure in response to the higher sodium diet. This led the authors to conclude that restricting sodium is particularly important in lowering blood pressure among more sedentary people. So, while we're better off watching our sodium, if you're active, maybe you can be a little more liberal with the salt. Perhaps knowing this might be a way to motivate people to exercise more!

Chapter 10

Seeing the Light at the End of the Tunnel: How Do We Get Out of This Mess?

It can be quite a challenge to eat a healthy diet these days. We live in an obesogenic environment, perfectly designed to foster food addiction. We have a food industry that is doing its best to maximize the hedonic value of the foods, to make them hyperpalatable, by tweaking the amount of sugar, salt, and fat they contain. Add in aggressive advertising and marketing, and it becomes very difficult to resist the temptation.

Personally, I do believe that the food industry should be held more accountable for the ways that their products impact our health and well-being. But if you ask a Food Giant executive, they will argue that their focus has to be to remain accountable to their shareholders. They need to continue to make "tasty" food in order to stay profitable. Why would they start down-formulating the usage of sugar, salt, and fat if the end result is going to be something that people do not want to eat, or buy?

But the good news is that we appear to be at a *tipping point* right now. The Food Giants are backed up against the wall. Some would say they're scared to death. On one hand, pressure from Wall Street for profits has never been greater. But, on the other hand, pressure from consumers for better, healthier products has also never been greater. How can they make and promote products that taste good, are profitable, but still healthy? How can they improve their image as well?

Meanwhile, there's pressure from the White House to do something to fight the escalating obesity crisis that's crippling our already fragile health care system. In June of 2013, the American Medical Association, for the first time, officially recognized obesity as a disease. The pediatric obesity crisis, in particular, has been receiving a lot of attention. And the landscape is definitely changing—gradually. For example, in November of 2006, the Council of Better Business Bureaus and leading food and beverage companies launched the *Children's Food and Beverage Advertising Initiative* (CFBAI), a voluntary, self-governing program created with the goal of shifting the mix of advertising directed primarily toward children (i.e., "child-directed advertising"). Their aim is to encourage healthier dietary choices and healthy lifestyles. Currently, the CFBAI has 17 participants that represent about 80 percent of all child-directed TV food advertising.

However, while such initiatives are certainly encouraging, a major factor that has yet to be fully addressed is cost. Cost is a huge issue in the big scheme of things. The food industry insists that processed foods, high in sugar, salt, and fat, are not demons, but rather safe, reliable, and cheap ways to deliver necessary calories. But others take an alternative view: the low cost of processed foods has actually been discouraging the development of healthier ways of feeding the world. According to

James Behnke, a former executive at Pillsbury, "We're hooked on inexpensive food, just like we're hooked on cheap energy." And, to make matters worse, when it comes to a quality diet, there's the growing disparity between the haves and have-nots. It simply costs more money to eat fresher, healthier foods. Sure, we can tell people to eat more fresh fruits and vegetables. But when you hit that grocery store and you see that a small basket of blueberries costs $5, whereas a large bag of chips or other processed foods, loaded with sugar, salt, and fat costs just a few bucks, what do you do? That's a really difficult dilemma for many households. How can a family on a budget manage to fill up their grocery cart for less money? Unfortunately, for many households, nutrition often takes a back seat. Many experts argue that it is for this reason that governmental regulation could be quite beneficial in leveling the playing field when it comes to the cost of eating well.

Putting such complicated issues aside, what can you do here and now to make a difference in your own lives, and in the lives of those who are in your sphere of influence?

1. **Get educated/spread the word.** By educating ourselves, our patients, clients, coworkers, families, friends, schools, neighbors, churches, and communities, we can learn what our bodies need to be healthy.

2. **Vote with your forks and wallets.** Your buying behavior can help keep the Food Giants accountable for the physical and social costs of their actions.

3. **Get a little louder.** As consumers, we must be louder with our concerns. We need to continue to put pressure on companies and government regulators to respond. With enough consumer and governmental pressure, food companies will need to react and produce more of the healthy foods we are demanding.

4. **Realize that we have power.** Yes, there are many forces taking place in the food industry, but, at

the same time, we need to realize that we are not helpless. We do have choices, particularly when it comes to grocery shopping. Knowing this can be empowering.

Michael Moss says:

> You can walk through the store and, while the brightly colored packaging and empty promises are mesmerizing, you can see the products for what they are. You can also see everything that goes on behind the image they project on the shelf: the formulas, the psychology, and the marketing that compels us to toss them in the cart. They may have salt, sugar, and fat on their side, but we, ultimately, have the power to make choices.[1]

5. **Set some nutritional goals to defend yourself against the onslaught of unhealthy foods.**

- lower your sweet threshold by limiting your consumption of refined carbs and added sugars

- choose *quality* carbohydrates that are high in fiber and have a low glycemic load

- eat less processed foods in general—foods with fewer ingredients, ingredients that you can pronounce

- when you do eat processed foods, consume less variety (variety promotes overeating)

- choose real, whole foods (those which your grandmother could recognize as food)

- choose higher quality fats (i.e., monounsaturated and omega-3 fatty acids)

- gradually reduce your sodium intake

6. **Examine your dependence on processed foods.** You might think that you simply can't stop eating processed foods. Part of the reason is that our lives are too busy, our kids are picky eaters, and many of us have taste buds that are still amped up from eating big doses of sugar, salt, and fat. So whether it's for convenience, pleasure, or just a matter of "getting by," we feel that we need our fix of Pop Tarts®, Kraft Macaroni & Cheese, Pringles, or Oreo cookies just to get through the day. But start

by making substitutions. Gradually decrease the number of processed foods that you eat. Think of the effect they are having on your body and brain. Get a little angry with the food industry. They are profiting at your expense.

7. **Be patient.** Your taste preferences will adjust. Certainly, what we like and dislike in food can and does change over time.[50] That means that your taste buds *can* get used to a healthier diet. Just be patient! Some experts suggest that it takes approximately 8 to 12 weeks to get used to a better quality diet. So, it may not be easy in the beginning. But stick with it! If we improve the quality of our diets and stay the course, we can reset our brain's reward circuitry and create a hedonic (perception of pleasure) shift. This means that, even though poor eating may have become a habit, if we practice better eating behaviors, we can essentially rewire our brains so that the healthier behaviors become as natural and as pleasant as the unhealthy behaviors they are replacing.

8. **Consider Food Rehab, if need be.** Gradually decreasing consumption of processed foods might sound fine for some, but for others who are struggling with a food addiction, the best approach might be to *avoid the offending food(s) altogether.* According to Dr. Nora Volkow, Director of the National Institute on Drug Abuse, overeating is as difficult to overcome as some drug addictions. She says:

> Clearly, processed sugar in certain individuals can produce compulsive patterns of intake. And, in those situations, I would recommend they just stay away. Don't try to limit yourself to two Oreo cookies because if the reward is very potent, no matter how good your intentions, you are not going to be able to control them—which is the same message we have for those addicted to drugs.

Dealing with a food addiction can be challenging. Perhaps you've heard it put this way: When you're addicted to drugs, you put the tiger in the cage to recover; when you're addicted to food, you put the tiger in the cage, but you have to take it out three times a day for a walk. Certainly you can't avoid food altogether, but you can avoid your "trigger" or "priming" foods. From a practical point of view, most foods that are a combination of high sugar and fat could be considered to be in the "danger zone." They are so stimulating, that many food addicts find it difficult to limit themselves to reasonable portions.

The next step is to work to reprogram your appetite. Learn to listen to your body and become a mindful eater. Focus on getting sufficient quality sleep, increasing your physical activity, and managing your stress. All these behaviors can help to bolster your physical resilience, improve appetite regulation, and reset your reward circuitry. Over time, once you've established new patterns and created a hedonic shift, you'll be able to once again open the doors to your favorite foods and determine whether they still act as triggers. You might be surprised, and relieved, to find that—over time—the foods that once held you captive are simply no longer all that appealing.

9. **Be a smarter shopper.** Here are some tips to consider:

- *Never shop without a list.* Some estimates suggest that about 60 percent of supermarket purchases are completely unplanned. Having a list helps to fend off the impulse to load up on sugary, salty, and fatty snacks. Have a list and stick to it.

- *Keep an educated eye out for sophisticating marketing techniques aimed at snagging you when you step foot in the store.* The industry's goal is to "engage the shopper early" with huge, eye-catching displays of poor quality food, right up front when there is maximum exposure and maximum traffic. Be smart. Have a critical eye. Don't fall prey to their tactics.

- *Shop primarily around the perimeter of the grocery store, where you are more likely to find real, whole foods.* Be aware that the center aisles are places where products that are heavily laden with sugar, salt, and fat are located.

- *Have your guard up at the check-out counter.*
  This is a prime spot for displaying soda and sugary foods. Stores take advantage of impulse-buying at the register. Don't get yourself in a situation where you are making spontaneous decisions to buy poor quality foods that are not on your list. Be strong.

- *When selecting particular food items, start by looking at the front of the packaging.* Look for claims such as: "low fat" and "low sugar" and "added calcium." These should be interpreted as warning signs. Products that state "low fat" are often loaded with sugar to make up for the reduction in fat. Likewise, products that are "low salt" are often loaded with sugar and fat to make up for the low salt. Just remember: "real food" doesn't have to rely on health claims. Next, look at the nutrition facts panel, which must be listed on most foods sold at retail stores, and on every package that makes a health claim. The information contained on that panel will reveal what *exactly* is in that package. And when you are examining the numbers, pay close attention to the number of servings per container. You may be surprised to find out that what you thought was a single serving, was actually calculated to feed four!

- *Be especially careful when shopping at convenience stores.* In addition to selling convenience, they focus on selling foods high in sugar, salt, and fat. Sometimes referred to as "C-stores," they are especially attractive to young kids and teens because they might be within a short distance to home or school, and sell single drinks and other affordable foods. The layout of C-stores is perfectly designed to grab our kids at every turn.

I hope that this book will help you to understand what the Food Giants are throwing at you in terms of formulations, marketing, and advertising. My goal is for you to feel more empowered to take control of your food choices, and to make choices that will ensure a healthier body and mind. Just remember that, in the end, you are the one who decides what to buy. You are the one who decides what to eat and how much. You hold that power.

References

1. Moss, Michael. *Salt, Sugar, Fat: How the Food Giants Hooked Us.* New York, NY: Random House, 2013.

2. Pollan, Michael. *In Defense of Food: An Eater's Manifesto.* Penguin Press: London, England, 2008.

3. Kessler DA. *The End of Overeating: Taking Control of The Insatiable American Appetite.* New York, NY: Rodale Books, 2009.

4. Simpson KA, Martin NM, Bloom SR. Hypothalamic regulation of appetite. *Expert Rev Endocrinol Metab.* 2008;3(5):577-592.

5. Berthoud HR. Metabolic and hedonic drives in the neural control of appetite: who is the boss? *Curr Opin Neurobiol.* 2011 Dec;21(6):888-896.

6. Lutter M, Nestler EJ. Homeostatic and hedonic signals interact in the regulation of food intake. *J Nutr.* 2009 Mar;139(3):629-632. Epub 2009 Jan 28. Review.

7. Pelchat ML. Of human bondage: food craving, obsession, compulsion and addiction. *Physiol. Behav.* 2002: 97:347-352.

8. Avena NM, Gold J, Kroll C, Gold S. Further Developments in the Neurobiology of Food and Addiction: Update on the State of the Science. *Nutrition.* 2012 April; 28(4):341-343.

9. Volkow ND, Wang G, Telang F. Cocaine Cues and Dopamine in Dorsal Striatum: Mechanism of Craving in Cocaine Addiction. *J Neurosci.* 2006; 26(4):6583-6588.

10. Drewnowski A, Krahn DD, Demitrack MA, Nairn K, Gosnell BA. Naloxone, an opiate blocker, reduces the consumption of sweet high-fat foods in obese and lean female binge eaters. *Am J Clin Nutr.* 1995. Jun;61(6):1206-1212.

11. Pelchat ML. Food addiction in humans. *J Nutr.* 2009 Mar;139(3):620-622.

12. Davis C, Carter JC. Compulsive overeating as an addiction disorder. A review of theory and evidence. *Appetite.* 2009 Aug;53(1):1-8.

13. American Psychiatric Association: *Diagnostic and Statistical Manual of Mental Disorders,* Fifth Edition. Arlington, VA: American Psychiatric Association, 2013.

14.   Gearhardt AN, Corbin WR, Brownell KD. Food Addiction: an examination of the diagnostic criteria for dependence. *J Addict Med.* 2009;3(1):1–7.

15.   Gearhardt AN, Yokum S, Orr PT, Stice E, Corbin WR, Brownell KD. Neural Correlates of Food Addiction. *Arch Gen Psychiat.* 2011 August;68(8):808-816.

16.   Stice E, Yokum S, Burger KS. Elevated reward region responsivity predicts future substance use onset but not overweight/obesity onset. *Biol Psychiatry.* 2013 May 1;73(9):869-876.

17.   Volkow ND, Wang GJ, Tomasi D, Baler RD. The addictive dimensionality of obesity. *Biol Psychiatry.* 2013 May 1;73(9):811-818. doi: 10.1016/j.biopsych.2012.12.020.

18.   Volkow ND, Wang GJ, Tomasi D. Pro v Con Reviews: Is Food Addictive? Obesity and addiction: neurobiological overlaps. *Obesity Reviews.* 2012;14:2-18.

19.   Volkow ND, Wang GJ, Fowler JS, et al. Overlapping neuronal circuits in addiction and obesity: evidence of systems pathology. *Philos Trans R Soc Lond B Biol Sci.* 2008 Oct 12;363(1507):3191-3200.

20.   Erlanson-Albertsson C. How palatable food disrupts appetite regulation. *Basic Clin Pharmacol Toxicol.* 2005;97:61-73.

21.   Johnson PM, Kenny PJ. Dopamine D2 receptors in addiction-like reward dysfunction and compulsive eating in obese rats. *Nat Neurosci.* 2010;13(5):635-641.

22.   Ifland JR, Preuss HG, Marcus MT, et al. Refined food addiction: a classic substance use disorder. *Med Hypotheses.* 2009 May;72(5):518-526.

23.   Thornley S, Russell B, Kydd R. Carbohydrate reward and psychosis: an explanation for neuroleptic induced weight gain and path to improved mental health? *Curr Neuropharmacol.* 2011 Jun;9(2):370-375.

24.   Parylak SL, Koob GF, Zorrilla EP. The dark side of food addiction. *Physiol Behav.* 2011 Jul 25;104(1):149-156.

25.   Iemolo A, Valenza M, Tozier L. et al. Withdrawal from chronic, intermittent access to a highly palatable food induces depressive-like behavior in compulsive eating rats. *Behav Pharmacol.* 2012 Sep;23(5-6):593-602.

References

26. Avena NM, Rada P, Hoebel BG. Sugar and fat bingeing have notable differences in addictive-like behavior. *J Nutr*. 2009 Mar;139(3):623-628.

27. Avena NM, Rada P, Hoebel BG. Evidence for sugar addiction: behavioral and neurochemical effects of intermittent, excessive sugar intake. *Neurosci Biobehav Rev*. 2008;32(1):20-39.

28. Stice E, Spoor S, Bohon C, SmallDM. Relation between obesity and blunted striatal response to food is moderated by *TaqIA* A1 allele. *Science*. 2008;322(5900):449-452.

29. Blum K, Bailey J, Gonzalez AM. Neuro-genetics of reward deficiency syn444drome as the root cause of "addiction transfer:" a new phenomenon common after bariatric surgery. *J Genet Syndr Gene Ther*. 2011 December 23;2012 (1):S2-001.

30. Avena NM, Gold J, Kroll C, Gold MS. Further developments in the neurobiology of food and addiction: update on the state of the science. *Nutrition*. 2012. April; 28(4):341-343).

31. CohenDA. Neurophysiological pathways to obesity: below awareness and beyond individual control. *Diabetes*. 2008;57:1768-1773.

32. Mattes RD, Popkin BM. Non-nutritive sweetener consumption in humans: Effects on appetite and food intake and their putative mechanisms. *Am J Clin Nutr*. 2009;89(1):1-14.

33. Wansink B. Environmental factors that increase the food intake and consumption volume of unknowing consumers. *Ann Rev Nutrition*. 2004;24:455-479.

34. Sclafani A, Springer D. Dietary obesity in adult rates: similarities to hypothalamic and human obesity syndromes. *Physiol Behav*. 1976; 17(3):461-471.

35. Katz D, Katz C. *The Flavor Point Diet: The Delicious Breakthrough Plan to Turn off Your Hunger and Lose the Weight for Good*. New York, NY: Rodale Books, 2005.

36. Rolls ET, et al. Sensory-specific satiety: Food-specific reduction in responsiveness of ventral forebrain neurons after feeding in the monkey. *Brain Res*.1986;368(1):79-86.

37. Wansink B. *Mindless Eating: Why We Eat More Than We Think*. New York, NY: Bantam Dell, 2006. www.mindlesseating.com. Assessed October 29, 2013.

38. Kahn BE, Wansink B. The influence of assortment structure on perceived variety and consumption quantities. *J Consumer Res.* 2004;30(4):519-533.

39. Rolls BJ. Experimental analyses of the effects of variety in a meal on human feeding. *Amer J Clin Nutrit.* 1985;42:932-939.

40. Pelchet ML, et al. Images of desire: food craving activation during fMRI. *Neuroimage.* 2004;23:1486-1493.

41. Burger KS, Stice E. Neuronal responsivity during soft drink intake, anticipation, and advertisement exposure in habitually consuming youth. *Obesity* (Silver Spring). 2013 July 9. doi: 10.1002/oby.20563) [Epub ahead of print]

42. Berthoud HR. The neurobiology of food intake in an obesogenic environment. *Proc Nutr Soc.* 2012;71(4):478-487.

43. Cantin L, Lenoir M, Augier E et al. Cocaine is low on the value ladder of rats: possible evidence for resilience to addiction. *PLoS One.* 2010;5:e11592.

44. Yarnell S, Oscar-Berman M, Avena N, . Pharmacotherapies for Overeating and Obesity. *J Genet Syndr Gene Ther.* 2013 Apr 1;4(3):131.

45. Garber AK, Lustig RH. Is fast food addictive? *Curr Drug Abuse Rev.* 2011 Sep 4(3):146-162.

46. Scrinis, Gyorgy. *Nutritionism: The Science and Politics of Dietary Advice.* Columbia University Press, Jackson, TN, June 2013. http://cup.columbia.edu/book/978-0-231-15656-1/nutritionism. Accessed October 29, 2013.

47. Nestle M. *Food Politics: How the Food Industry Influences Nutrition and Health.* Berkeley, CA: University of California Press, 2000.

48. Campbell, T Collins. *Whole: Rethinking the Science of Nutrition.* Dallas, TX: BenBella Books, 2013.

49. Scrinis G. On the ideology of nutritionalism. *Gastronomica: the journal of food and culture.* Winter 2008;8:(1):39–48. Issn 1529-3262.

50. Pelletier, C. Beyond the Tongue Map: Evaluating Taste and Smell Perception. *The ASHA Leader.* October 22, 2002.

References

51. Sclafani A, Glass DS, Margolskee RF. Gut T1R3 sweet taste receptors do not mediate sucrose-conditioned flavor preferences in mice. *Am J Physiol Regul Integr Comp Physiol.* 2010 Dec;299(6):R1643-R1650.

52. Yee KK, Sukumaran SK, Kotha R, et al. Glucose transporters and ATP-gated K (KATP) metabolic sensors are present in type 1 taste receptor 3 (T1r3)-expressing taste cells. *Proc Natl Acad Sci.* 2011 March 29;108(13):5431-5436, DOI:10.1073/pnas.1100495108

53. Yudkin J. *Pure, white and deadly: the problem of sugar.* London, UK: Viking Press, 1986.

54. Johnson RK, Appel LJ, Brands M, et al. Dietary sugars intake and cardiovascular health: a scientific statement from the American Heart Association. *Circulation.* August 2009;120(11):1011-1120. [Epub 2009 August 24]

55. United States Department of Agriculture. *2010 Dietary Guidelines for Americans.* www.DietaryGuidelines.gov. Accessed October 29, 2013.

56. National Cancer Institute. Usual intake of added sugars. In: *Usual Dietary Intakes: Food Intakes, US Population 2001–04.* November 2008. http://riskfactor.cancer.gov/diet/usualintakes/pop/. Accessed October 29, 2013.

57. Ervin RS, Kit BK, Carroll MD, et al. Consumption of added sugar among US children and adolescents, 205-2998. *NCHS Data Brief.* 2012 March;87:1-8.

58. Malik VS. Popkin BM, Bray GA, et al. Sugar-sweetened beverages, obesity, type 2 diabetes mellitus, and cardiovascular disease risk. *Circulation.* 2010 Mar;121:1356-1364.

59. Briefel RR, Johnson CL. Secular trends in dietary intake in the United States. *Ann Rev Nutr.* 2004;24:401-431.

60. Nielsen SJ, Siega-Riz AM, Popkin BM. Trends in energy intake in U.S. between 1977 and 1996: similar shifts seen across age groups. *Obes Res.* 2002;10:370-378.

61. US Department of Agriculture. MyPlate. Updated August 15, 2013. http://www.cnpp.usda.gov/MyPlate.htm. Accessed October 29, 2013.

62. Nielson SJ, Popkin BM. Changes in beverage intake between 1977 and 2001. *Am J Prev Med.* 2004;27(3):205-210.

63. Ludwig DS, Peterson KE, Gortmaker SL. Relation between consumption of sugar-sweetened drinks and childhood obesity: a prospective, observational analysis. *Lancet.* 2001;357:505-508.

64. Schulze MB, Manson JE, Ludwig DS, et al. Sugar-sweetened beverages, weight gain, and incidence of type 2 diabetes in young and middle-aged women. *JAMA.* 2004;292(8):927-934;978-979.

65. McKiernan F, Houchins JA, Mattes RD. Relationships between human thirst, hunger, drinking, and feeding. *Physiol Behav.* 2008 Aug 6;94(5):700-708. [Epub 2008 Apr 13]

66. Brownell KD, Farley T, Willett WC. The public health and economic benefits of taxing sugar-sweetened beverages. *N Engl J Med.* 2009;361(16):1599-1605.

67. Bremer AA, Auinger P, Byrd RS. Relationship between insulin resistance-associated metabolic parameters and anthropometric measurements with sugar-sweetened beverage intake and physical activity levels in US adolescents: Findings from the 1999-2004 National Health and Nutrition Examination Survey. *Arch Pediatr Adolesc Med.* 2009;163(4):328-335.

68. Welsh JA, Sharma A, Abramson JL. Caloric sweetener consumption and dyslipidemia among US adults. *JAMA.* 2010;303(15):1490-1497.

69. Perez-Pozo SE, Schold J, Nakagawa T, et al. Excessive fructose intake induces the features of metabolic syndrome in healthy adult men: role of uric acid in the hypertensive response. *Inter J Obes Relat Metab Disord.* 2009;34:454-461.

70. Welsh JA, et al. Consumption of Added Sugars and Indicators of Cardiovascular Disease Risk Among US Adolescents. *Circulation.* 2011;123:249-257.

71. Dhingra R, Sullivan L, Jacques PF, Wang TJ, et al. Soft drink consumption and risk of developing cardiometabolic risk factors and the metabolic syndrome in middle-aged adults in the community. *Circulation.* 2007;116:480-488.

72. Winkelmayer WC, Stampfer MJ, Willett WC, Curhan GC. Habitual caffeine intake and the risk of hypertension in women. *JAMA.* 2005;294:2330-2335.

References

73. Brown IJ, Stamler J, Van Horn L, et al. Sugar-sweetened beverage, sugar intake of individuals and their blood pressure: International Study of micro/macronutrients and blood pressure. *Hypertension.* 2011 Apr;57(4):695-701.

74. Choi JW, Ford ES, Gao X, Choi HK. Sugar-sweetened soft drinks, diet soft drinks, and serum uric acid level: the Third National Health and Nutrition Examination Survey. *Arthritis Rheum.* 2008;59:109-116.

75. Choi HK, Curhan G. Soft drinks, fructose consumption, and the risk of gout in men: prospective cohort study. *BMJ.* 2008;336:309–312.

76. Fung TT, Malik V, Rexrode KM, Manson JE, Willett WC, Hu FB. Sweetened beverage consumption and risk of coronary heart disease in women. *Am J Clin Nutr.* 2009;89:1037–1042.

77. Mosca L, Benjamin EJ, Berra K, et al. Effectiveness-based guidelines for the prevention of cardiovascular disease in women—2011 update. A guideline from the American Heart Association. *Circulation.* 2011;23:1243-1262.

77.1 Oswald KD, Murdaugh DL, King VL. Motivation for palatable food despite consequences in an animal model of binge eating. *Int J Eat Disord.* 2010 doi: 10.1002/eat.20808.

78. Lennerz BS, Alsop DC, Holsen LM, et al. Effects of dietary glycemic index on brain regions related to reward and craving in men. *Am J Clin Nutrition.* 2013 Sept;98(3):641-647.

79. Shelton RC, Miller AH. Inflammation in depression: is adiposity a cause? *Dialogues Clin Neurosci.* 2011;13(1):41-53.

80. Nakagawa T, Zharikov S, et al. A causal role for uric acid in fructose-induced metabolic syndrome. *Am J Physiol Renal Physiol.* 2006;290:F625-F631.

81. Jalal DI, Smits G, Johnson RJ, et al. Increased fructose associates with elevated blood pressure. *J Am Soc Neprhol.* July 2010;21(9)1543-1549.

82. Bantle JP. Dietary fructose and metabolic syndrome and diabetes. *J Nutr.* 2009 June;139(6):1263S-1268S.

83. Lê KA, Tappy L. Metabolic effects of fructose. *Curr Opin Clin Nutr Metab Care.* 2006;9:469-475.

84. Havel PJ. Dietary fructose: implications for dysregulation of energy homeostasis and lipid/carbohydrate metabolism. *Nutr Rev.* 2005;63:133-157.

85. Gross LS, Li S, Ford ES, Liu S. Increased consumption of refined carbohydrates and the epidemic of type 2 diabetes in the United States: an ecologic assessment. *Am J Clin Nutr.* 2004;79:774-779.

86. Elliott SS, Keim NL, Stern JS, Teff K, Havel PJ. Fructose, weight gain, and the insulin resistance syndrome. *Am J Clin Nutr.* 2002;76:911-922.

87. White JS, Foreyt JP, Melanson KJ, et al. High-fructose corn syrup: controversies and common sense. *Am J Lifestyle Med.* 2010;4(6):515-520 .

88. Rizkalla SW. Health implications of fructose consumption: A review of recent data. *Nutr Metab* (Lond). 2010;7:82.

89. Dolan LC, Potter SM, Burdock GA. Evidence-based review on the effect of normal dietary consumption of fructose on development of hyperlipidemia and obesity in healthy, normal weight individuals. *Crit Rev Food Sci Nutr.* 2010;50:53-84.

90. Tappy L, Le KA. Metabolic effects of fructose and the worldwide increase in obesity. *Physiol Rev.* 2010;90:23-46.

91. Page KA, CHAN O, Arora J. et al. Effects of Fructose vs Glucose on Regional Cerebral Blood Flow in Brain Regions Involved With Appetite and Reward Pathways. *JAMA.* 2013;309(1):63-70.

92. Pimentel GD, Micheletti TO, et al. Gut-central nervous system axis is a target for nutritional therapies. *Nutr J.* 2012;11:22.

93. Jeffery IB, O'Toole PW. Diet-microbiota interactions and their implications for healthy living. *Nutrients.* 2013 Jan 17;5(1):234-252. doi: 10.3390/nu5010234.

94. Payne AN, Chassard C, Lacroix C. Gut microbial adaptation to dietary consumption of fructose, artificial sweeteners and sugar alcohols: implications for host-microbe interactions contributing to obesity. *Obes Rev.* 2012 Sep;13(9):799-809.

95. Kanoski SE, Davidson TL. Western Diet Consumption and Cognitive Impairment: Links to Hippocampal Dysfunction and Obesity. *Physiol Behav.* 2011 April 18; 103(1):59-68.

References

96. Bosma-den Boer MM, van Wetten ML, Pruimboom L. Chronic inflammatory diseases are stimulated by current lifestyle: how diet, stress levels and medication prevent our body from recovering. *Nutr Metab* (Lond). 2012 Apr 17;9(1):32.

97. Kiecolt-Glaser, J. Stress, food, & inflammation: psychoneuroimmunology and nutrition at the cutting edge. *Psychosom Med.* 2010;72(4):365-369.

98. Baskin DG et al. Insulin signaling in the central nervous system. *Diabetes.* 2005;54:1264-1276.

99. Craft S. The role of metabolic disorders in Alzheimers disease and vascular dementia: two roads converged? *Arch Neurol.* 2009;66(3):300-305.

100. Agrawal R., Gomez-Pinilla F. 'Metabolic syndrome' in the brain: deficiency in omega-3 fatty acid exacerbates dysfunctions in insulin receptor signalling and cognition. *J Physiol.* 2012 May 15;590:2485-2499.

101. Position of the American Dietetic Association: Use of nutritive and nonnutritive sweeteners. *J Am Dietetic Assoc.* 2004;104:255-275.

102. Schulze MB, Manson JE, Ludwig DS, et al. Sugar-sweetened beverages, weight gain, and incidence of type 2 diabetes in young and middle-aged women. *JAMA.* 2004;292(8):927-934.

103. Tordoff MG, Alleva AM. Effect of drinking soda sweetened with aspartame or high-fructose corn syrup on food intake and body weight. *Am J Clin Nutr.* 1990;51(6):963-969.

104. Raben A, Vasilaras TH, Moller AC, et al. Sucrose compared with artificial sweeteners: different effects on ad libitum food intake and body weight after 10 wk of supplementation in overweight subjects. *Am J Clin Nutr.* 2002;76(4):721-729.

105. Blackburn GL, Kanders BS, Lavin PT, et al. The effect of aspartame as part of a multidisciplinary weight-control program on short- and long-term control of body weight. *Am J Clin Nutr.* 1997;65(2):409-418.

106. Mattes RD, Popkin BM. Non-nutritive sweetener consumption in humans: Effects on appetite and food intake and their putative mechanisms. *Am J Clin Nutr.* 2009 January;89(1):1-14.

107. Fowler SP, Williams K, Resendez RG, et al. Fueling the obesity epidemic? Artificially sweetened beverage use and long-term weight gain. *Obesity*. 2008;16(8):1894-1900.

108. Lutsey PL, Steffen LM, Stevens J. Dietary intake and the development of the metabolic syndrome: the Atherosclerosis Risk in Communities study. *Circulation*. 2008;117(6):754-761.

109. Dhingra R, Sullivan L, Jacques PF, et al. Soft drink consumption and risk of developing cardiometabolic risk factors and the metabolic syndrome in middle-aged adults in the community. *Circulation*. 2007;116(5):480-488.

110. Winkelmayer WC, Stampfer MJ, Willett WC, et al. Habitual caffeine intake and the risk of hypertension in women. *JAMA*. 2005;294(18):2330-2335.

111. Nettleton JA, Lutsey PL, Wang Y, et al. Diet soda intake and risk of incident metabolic syndrome and type 2 diabetes in the Multi-Ethnic Study of Atherosclerosis (MESA). *Diabetes Care*. 2009;32(4):688-694.

112. Brown RJ, De Banate MA, Rother KI. Artificial Sweeteners: A systematic review of metabolic effects in youth. *Int J Pediatr Obes*. 2010 August;5(4):305-312.

113. Swithers SE, Davidson TL. A role for sweet taste: calorie predictive relations in energy regulation by rats. *Behav Neurosci*. 2008 Feb;122(1):161-173.

114. Swithers, Susan E. Artificial sweeteners produce the counterintuitive effect of inducing metabolic derangements. *Trends Endocrinol Metabol*. [Epun July 10, 2013]

115. Mace OJ, Affleck J, Patel N, et al. Sweet taste receptors in rat small intestine stimulate glucose absorption through apical GLUT2. *J Physiol*. 2007;582(Pt 1):379-392.

116. Brown RJ, Rother K Non-nutritive sweeteners and their role in the gastrointestinal tract. *J Clin Endocrinol Metab*. 2012 Aug;97(8):2597-605. doi: 10.1210/jc.2012-1475.[Epub 2012 Jun 7]

117. Dyer J, Salmon KS, Zibrik L, et al. Expression of sweet taste receptors of the T1R family in the intestinal tract and enteroendocrine cells. *Biochem Soc Trans*. 2005;33(Pt 1):302-305.

References

118. Margolskee RF, Dyer J, Kokrashvili Z, et al. T1R3 and gustducin in gut sense sugars to regulate expression of Na+-glucose cotransporter 1. *Proc Natl Acad Sci USA.* 2007;104(38):15075-15080.

119. Jang HJ, Kokrashvili Z, Theodorakis MJ, et al. Gut-expressed gustducin and taste receptors regulate secretion of glucagonlike peptide-1. *Proc Natl Acad Sci USA.* 2007;104(38):15069-15074.

120. Brown RJ, Walter M, Rother KI. Ingestion of diet soda before a glucose load augments glucagon-like peptide-1. *Diab Care.* 2009;32(12):2184-2186.

121. Pepino MY, Tiemann CD, Patterson BW, et al. Sucralose affects glycemic and hormonal response to an oral glucose load. *Diab Care.* [Epub April 30, 2013]

122. Pepino MY, Bourne C. Non-nutritive sweeteners, energy balance, and glucose homeostasis. *Curr Opin Clin Nutr Metab Care.* 2011 Jul;14(4):391-395.

123. Olney JW, Ho OL. Brain damage in infant mice following oral intake of glutamate, aspartate or cysteine. *Nature.* 1970;227:609-611.

124. Schainker B, Olney JW. Glutamate-type hypothalamic-pituitary syndrome in mice treated with aspartate or cysteate in infancy. *J Neural Transm.* 1974;35:207-215.

125. Gardner C, Wylie-Rosett J, Gidding SS, et al. Nonnutritive sweeteners: Current use and health perspectives. A scientific statement from the American Heart Association and the American Diabetes Association. *Circulation.* 2012; 126:509-519.

126. Gardner C, Wylie-Rosett J, Gidding SS, et al. Nonnutritive sweeteners: Current use and health perspectives. A scientific statement from the American Heart Association and the American Diabetes Association. *Diabetes Care.* 2012 Jul 24;126(4):509-519. DOI:10.2337/dc12-9002. .

127. David Mendosa. Mendosa.com. Revised International Table of Glycemic Index (GI) and Glycemic Load (GL) Values—2002. http://www.mendosa.com/gilists.htm. Accessed October 29, 2013.

128. Abdel-Rahman A, Anyangwe N, Carlacci L, et al. The safety and regulation of natural products used as foods and food ingredients. *Toxicol Sci.* 2011 Oct;123(2):333-348.

129. Goyal SK, Samsher, Goay RK. Stevia (Stevia rebaudiana) a bio-sweetener: a review. *Int J Food SciNutr.* 2010 Feb;61(1):1-10.

130. Van Oudenhove L, McKie S, Lassman D, et al.. Fatty acid-induced gut-brain signaling attenuates neural and behavioral effects of sad emotion in humans. *J Clin Invest.* 2011 Aug;121(8):3094-3099.

131. Cizza G, Rother KI. Was Feuerbach right: are we what we eat? *J Clin Invest.* 2011 Aug;121(8):2969-2971.

132. Bocarsly ME, Berner LA, Hoebel BG, Avena NM. Rats that binge eat fat-rich food do not show somatic signs or anxiety associated with opiate-like withdrawal: Implications for nutrient-specific food addiction behaviors. *Physiol Behav.* 2011 Oct 24;104(5):865-872.

133. Avena NM, Bocarsly ME, Rada P, Kim A, Hoebel BG. After daily bingeing on a sucrose solution, food deprivation induces anxiety and accumbens dopamine/acetylcholine imbalance. *Physiol Behav.* 2008 Jun 9;94(3):309–315.

134. Colantuoni C, Rada P, McCarthy J, Patten C, Avena NM, Chadeayne A, et al. Evidence that intermittent, excessive sugar intake causes endogenous opioid dependence. *Obes Res.* 2002 Jun;10(6):478–488.

135. Huth PJ, Park KM. Influence of dairy product and milk fat consumption on cardiovascular disease risk: a review of the evidence. *Adv Nutr.* 2012 May 1;3(3):266-285. doi: 10.3945/an.112.002030.

136. Lawrence GD. Dietary fats and health: Dietary recommendations in the context of scientific evidence. *Adv Nutr.* 2013; 4:294-302.

137. Siri-Tarino PW, Sun Q, Hu FB. Meta-analysis of prospective cohort studies evaluating the association of saturated fat with cardiovascular disease. *Am J Clin Nutr.* 2010; 91(3):535-546.

138. Galgani JE. Effect of dietary fat quality on insulin sensitivity. *Br J Nutr.* 2008;100(3):471-479.

139. Risérus U, Willett WC, Hu FB. Dietary fats and prevention of type 2 diabetes. *Prog Lipid Res.* 2009;48(1):44-51.

140. Benoit SC, Kemp CJ, Abplanalp W, et al. Palmitic acid mediates hypothalamic insulin resistance by altering PKC-θ subcellular localization in rodents. *J Clin Invest.* 2009;119(9):2577-2589.

References

141. Sharma MD, Garber AJ, Farmer JA. Role of insulin signaling in maintaining energy homeostasis. *Endocr Pract.* 2008;14(3):373-380. Review.

142. Morris M, Evans D, Tangney C, et al.. Dietary copper and high saturated and trans fat intakes associated with cognitive decline. *Arch Neurol.* 2006;63:1085–1088.

143. Morris MC, et al. Dietary fats and the risk of incident Alzheimer disease. *Arch Neurol.* 2003;60:194–200.

144. Kanoski SE, Davidson TL. Western Diet Consumption and Cognitive Impairment: Links to Hippocampal Dysfunction and Obesity. *Physiol Behav.* 2011 April 18;103(1):59-68.

145. Hanson AJ, Bayer-Carter JL, Green PS, et al. Effect of Apolipoprotein E Genotype and Diet on Apolipoprotein E Lipidation and Amyloid Peptides. *JAMA Neurol.* 2013;70(8):972-980. doi:10.1001/jamaneurol.2013.396.

146. Wen H, Gris D, Lei Y, et al. Fatty acid–induced NLRP3-ASC inflammasome activation interferes with insulin signaling. *Nature Immunology.* 2011;12:408–415.

147. L'homme L, Esser N, Riva L et al.Unsaturated fatty acids prevent activation of NLRP3 inflammasome in human monocytes/macrophages. *J Lipid Res.* 2013 Nov;54:2998-3008.

148. Stienstra R, Tack CJ, Kanneganti TD, The inflammasome puts obesity in the danger zone. *Cell Metab.* 2012 Jan 4;15(1):10-8. doi: 10.1016/j.cmet.2011.10.011.

149. Lamkanfi M, Walle LV, Kanneganti TD. Deregulated inflammasome signaling in disease. *Immunol Rev.* 2011 Sep;243(1):163-73. doi: 10.1111/j.1600-065X.2011.01042.x.

150. Lukens JR, Dixit VD, Kanneganti TD. Inflammasome activation in obesity-related inflammatory diseases and autoimmunity. *Discov Med.* 2011 Jul;12(62):65-74.

151. Iggman D, Risérus U. Role of Different Dietary Saturated Fatty Acids for Cardiometabolic Risk. *Clin Lipidology.* 2011;6(2):209-223.

152. Mensink RP, Katan MB: Effect of dietary fatty acids on serum lipids and lipoproteins. *Arterioscl Throm Vas.* 1992, 12:911-919.

153. Mensink RP, Zock PL, Kester AD, Katan MB: Effects of dietary fatty acids and carbohydrates on the ratio of serum total HDL cholesterol and on serum lipids and apolipoproteins: A meta-analysis of 60 controlled trials. *Am J Clin Nutr.* 2003, 77:1146-55.

154. Kris-Etherton PMYS: Individual fatty acid effects on plasma lipids and lipoproteins. Human studies. *Am J Clin Nutr.* 1997, 65(suppl.5):1628S-1644S.

155. Huth PJ, Park KM. Influence of dairy product and milk fat consumption on cardiovascular disease risk: a review of the evidence. *Adv Nutr.* 2012 May 1;3(3):266-285. doi: 10.3945/an.112.002030

156. Feranil AB, Duazo PL, Kuzawa CW, Adair LS. Coconut oil predicts a beneficial lipid profile in pre-menopausal women in the Philippines. *Asia Pac J Clin Nutr.* 2011;20(2):190–195.

157. Prior I, Davidson F, Salmond C, Czochanska Z. Cholesterol, coconuts and diet on Polynesian atolls: a natural experiment: The Pukapula and Tokelau Island Studies. *Am J Clin Nutr.* 1981;34:1442-1461.

158. Dayrit C. Coconut Oil: Atherogenic or Not? (What therefore causes atherosclerosis?) *Philipp J Cardiol.* 2003;31(3):97-104.

159. Rego Costa AC, Rosado EL, Soares-Mota M Influence of the dietary intake of medium chain triglycerides on body composition, energy expenditure and satiety: a systematic review. *Nutr Hosp.* 2012 Jan-Feb;27(1):103-8. doi: 10.1590/S0212-16112012000100011.

160. Newport, MT. *Alzheimer's Disease: What If There Was a Cure? The Story of Ketones.* Lagguna Beach CA: Basic Health Publications, 2011.

161. Daviglus ML, Bell CC, Berrettini W, et al. National Institutes of Health State-of-the-Science Conference statement: preventing Alzheimer disease and cognitive decline. *Ann Intern Med.* 2010;153:176-181.

162. McPherson PA, McEneny J. The biochemistry of ketogenesis and its role in weight management, neurological disease and oxidative stress. *J Physiol Biochem.* 2012;68:141-151.

163. Sacks FM, Katan M: Randomized clinical trials on the effects of dietary fat and carbohydrate on plasma lipoproteins and cardiovascular disease. *Am J Med.* 2002;113(Suppl. 9B):13S–24S.

164. Huth PJ, Park KM. Influence of dairy product and milk fat consumption on cardiovascular disease risk: a review of the evidence. *Adv Nutr.* 2012 May 1;3(3):266-285. doi: 10.3945/an.112.002030

165. Kratz M, Baars T, Guyenet S. The relationship between high-fat dairy consumption and obesity, cardiovascular, and metabolic disease. *Eur J Nutr.* 2013 Feb;52(1):1-24.

166. Lamarche B: Review of the effect of dairy products on non-lipid risk factors for cardiovascular disease. *J Am Coll Nutr.* 2008;27:741S–746S.

167. Zemel MB. The role of dairy foods in weight management. *J Am Coll Nutr.* 2005;24:537S–546S.

168. Ditscheid B, Keller S, Jahreis G: Cholesterol metabolism is affected by calcium phosphate supplementation in humans. *J Nutr.* 2005;135:1678–1682.

169. Tholstrup T, Hoy CE, Andersen LN, Christensen RD, Sandstrom B. Does fat in milk, butter and cheese affect blood lipids and cholesterol differently? *J Am Coll Nutr.* 2004;23:169-176.

170. Werner LB, Hellgren LI, Raff M, et al. Effects of butter from mountain-pasture grazing cows on risk markers of the metabolic syndrome compared with conventional Danish butter: a randomized controlled study. *Lipids Health Dis.* 2013 Jul 10;12:99. doi: 10.1186/1476-511X-12-99

171. Ludwig DS, Willett WC. Three daily servings of reduced-fat milk: an evidence based recommendation. *JAMA Pediatr.* 2013:167(9):788-789.

172. Key TJ. Diet, insulin-like growth factor-1 and cancer risk. *Proc Nutr Soc.* 2011 May 3:1-4. [Epub ahead of print]

173. Mozaffarian D, Micha R, Wallace S. Effects on coronary heart disease of increasing polyunsaturated fat in place of saturated fat: a systematic review and meta-analysis of randomized controlled trials. *PLoS Med.* 2010 Mar 23;7(3):e1000252.

174. Micha R, Mozaffarian D: Trans fatty acids: effects on cardiometabolic health and implications for policy. *Prostaglandins Leuko Essent Fatty Acids.* 2008;79:147-152.

175. Dorfman SE, Laurent D, Gounarides JS, et al. Metabolic implications of dietary trans-fatty acids. *Obesity (Silver Spring)*. 2009 Jun;17(6):1200-1207.

176. Tardy AL, Morio B, Chardigny JM, Malpuech-Brugère C. Ruminant and industrial sources of trans-fat and cardiovascular and diabetic diseases. *Nutr Res Rev.* 2011;15:1-7.

177. Sánchez-Villegas A, Verberne L, De Irala J, Ruíz-Canela M, Toledo E, et al. 2011 Dietary Fat Intake and the Risk of Depression: The SUN Project. *PLoS ONE.* 2011;6(1):e16268.

178. Gillingham LG, Harris-Janz S, Jones PJ. Dietary monounsaturated Fatty acids are protective against metabolic syndrome and cardiovascular disease risk factors. *Lipids.* 2011 Mar;46(3):209-228.

179. Schwingshackl L, Hoffmann G. Monounsaturated fatty acids and risk of cardiovascular disease: synopsis of the evidence available from systematic reviews and meta-analyses. *Nutrients.* 2012 Dec 11;4(12):1989-2007. doi: 10.3390/nu4121989

180. Attya M, Benabdelkamel H, Perri E, Effects of conventional heating on the stability of major olive oil phenolic compounds by tandem mass spectrometry and isotope dilution assay. *Molecules.* 2010 Dec 1;15(12):8734-8746. doi: 10.3390/molecules15128734.

181. Rafehi H, Ververis K, Karagiannis TC. Mechanisms of action of phenolic compounds in olive. *J Diet Suppl.* 2012 Jun;9(2):96-109. doi: 10.3109/19390211.2012.682644

182. Shai I, Schwarzfuchs D, Hankin R, et al. Dietary intervention randomized controlled trial. Weight loss with a carbohydrate, Mediterranean, or low-fat diet. *New Engl J Medicine.* 2008;359(3):229-241.

183. Pauwels EK. The protective effect of the Mediterranean diet: focus on cancer and cardiovascular risk. *Med Princ Pract.* 2011;20(2):103-111.

184. Simopoulos AP. The Mediterranean diets: What is so special about the diet of Greece? The scientific evidence. *J Nutr.* 2001 Nov;131(11 Suppl):3065S-3073S.

185. Sánchez-Villegas A, Delgado-Rodríguez M, Alonso A, et al. Association of the Mediterranean dietary pattern with the incidence of depression. *Arch Gen Psychiatry.* 2009;66(10):1090-1098.

References

186. Ramsden CE, Zamora D, Leelarthaepin B. et al. Use of Dietary Linoleic Acid for Secondary Prevention of Coronary Heart Disease and Death: Evaluation of Recovered Data From the Sydney Diet Heart Study and Updated Meta-Analysis. *BMJ.* 2013;346:e8707.

187. Brookes, L, Ramsden CE. The PUFA Investigation: An Expert Interview. Medscape Cardiology: Best Evidence Interviews in Cardiology. Mar 18, 2013. http://www.medscape.com/viewarticle/780949. Accessed October 29, 2013.

188. He K, Song Y, Daviglus ML, et al. Accumulated evidence on fish consumption and coronary heart disease mortality: a meta-analysis of cohort studies. *Circulation.* 2004;109:2705-2711.

189. US Environmental Protection Agency. Food and Drug Administration/ Center for Food Safety and Applied Nutrition. *Mercury study report to Congress.* http://www.epa.gov/hg/report.htm. Accessed October 29, 2013.

190. Kris-Etherton PM, Harris WS, Appel LJ. American Heart Association Nutrition Committee. Fish consumption, fish oil, omega-3 fatty acids, and cardiovascular disease. *Circulation.* 2002;106:2747-2757.

191. Makhoul Z, Kristal AR, Gulati R. Associations of obesity with triglycerides and C-reactive protein are attenuated in adults with high red blood cell eicosapentaenoic and docosahexaenoic acids. *Euro J Clin Nutr.* 2011 July;65(7):808-817.

192. Mozaffarian D, Lemaitre RN, Kuller LH, Burke GL, Tracy RP, Siscovick DS. Cardiovascular Health Study. Cardiac benefits of fish consumption may depend on the type of fish meal consumed: The Cardiovascular Health Study. *Circulation.* 2003 Mar 18;107(10):1372-1377,

193. Goyens PL, Spilker ME, Zock PL, et al. Conversion of α-linolenic acid in humans is influenced by the absolute amounts of α-linolenic acid and linoleic acid in the diet and not by their ratio. *Am J Clin Nutr.* 2006;84(1):44-53.

194. Risk and Prevention Study Collaborative Group, Roncaglioni MC, Tombesi M, et al. n-3 fatty acids in patients with multiple cardiovascular risk factors. *N Engl J Med.* 2013;368:1800-1808.

195. Kotwal S, Jun M, Sullivan D, Perkovic V, Neal B. Omega 3 fatty acids and cardiovascular outcomes: systematic review and meta-analysis. *Circ Cardiovasc Qual Outcomes.* 2012;5:808-818.

196. Rizos EC, Ntzani EE, Bika E, Kostapanos MS, Elisaf MS. Association between omega-3 fatty acid supplementation and risk of major cardiovascular disease events: a systematic review and meta-analysis. *JAMA*. 2012;308:1024-1033.

197. Manson JE, Bassuk SS, Lee IM, et al. The VITamin D and OmegA-3 TriaL (VITAL): rationale and design of a large randomized controlled trial of vitamin D and marine omega-3 fatty acid supplements for the primary prevention of cancer and cardiovascular disease. *Contemp Clin Trials*. 2012;33:159-171.

198. Sathyanarayana R, Ahsa , Ramesh BN, Jagannatha Rao KS. Understanding nutrition, depression and mental illnesses. *Indian J Psychiatry*. 2008 Apr;50(2):77-82.

199. Gow RV, Matsudaira T, Taylor E, et al. Total red blood cell concentrations of omega-3 fatty acids are associated with emotion-elicited neural activity in adolescent boys with attention-deficit hyperactivity disorder. *Prostaglandins Leukot Essent Fatty Acids*. 2009 Feb-Mar;80(2-3):151-156.

200. Turnbull T, Cullen-Drill M, Smaldone A. Efficacy of omega-3 fatty acid supplementation on improvement of bipolar symptoms: a systematic review. *Arch Psychiatr Nurs*. 2008;22:305–311.

201. Amminger GP, Schafer MR, Papageorgiou K, Klier CM, Cotton SM, et al. Long-chain omega-3 fatty acids for indicated prevention of psychotic disorders: a randomized, placebo-controlled trial. *Arch Gen Psychiatry*. 2010;67:146–154.

202. Richardson AJ. Omega-3 fatty acids in ADHD and related neurodevelopmental disorders. *Int Rev Psychiatry*. 2006;18:155–172.

203. Sarris J, Mischoulon D, Schweitzer I. Omega-3 for bipolar disorder: meta-analyses of use in mania and bipolar depression. *J Clin Psychiatry*. 2012;73:81–86.

204. Sublette ME, Ellis SP, Geant AL, Mann JJ. Meta-analysis of the effects of eicosapentaenoic acid (EPA) in clinical trials in depression. *J Clin Psychiatry*. 2011;72:1577–1584.

205. Fusar-Poli P, Berger G. Eicosapentaenoic acid interventions in schizophrenia: meta-analysis of randomized, placebo-controlled studies. *J Clin Psychopharmacol*. 2012;32:179-185.

References

206. Ortega RM, Rodriguez-Rodriguez E, Lopez-Sobaler AM. Effects of omega-3 fatty acids supplementation in behavior and non-neurodegenerative neuropsychiatric disorders. *Brit J Nutr.* 2012; 107(Suppl):2S261–2S270.

207. Freeman MP, Hibbeln JR, Wisner KL, et al. Omega-3 fatty acids: evidence basis for treatment and future research in psychiatry. *J Clin Psychiatry.* 2006;67:1954–1967.

208. Koletzko B, Lien E, Agostoni C, World Association of Perinatal Medicine Dietary Guidelines Working Group. The roles of long-chain polyunsaturated fatty acids in pregnancy, lactation and infancy: review of current knowledge and consensus recommendations. *J Perinat Med.* 2008;36(1):5-14.

209. Montgomery P, Burton JR, Sewell RP, Spreckelsen TF, Richardson AJ. Low Blood Long Chain Omega-3 Fatty Acids in UK Children Are Associated with Poor Cognitive Performance and Behavior: A Cross-Sectional Analysis from the DOLAB Study. *PLoS ONE.* 2013;8(6):e66697.

210. Narendran R, Frankle WG, Mason NS, Muldoon MF, Moghaddam B. Improved Working Memory but No Effect on Striatal Vesicular Monoamine Transporter Type 2 after Omega-3 Polyunsaturated Fatty Acid Supplementation. *PLoS ONE.* 2012;7(10):e46832.

211. Gestuvo MK, Hung WW. Common dietary supplements for cognitive health. *Aging Health.* 2012;8(1):89-97.

212. Mazereeuw G, Lanctôt KL, Chau SA, Swardfager W, Herrmann N. Effects of omega-3 fatty acids on cognitive performance: a meta-analysis. *Neurobiol Aging.* 2012;33:1482.e17-e29.

213. Villani AM, Crotty M, Cleland LG Fish oil administration in older adults: is there potential for adverse events? A systematic review of the literature. *BMC Geriatr.* 2013 May 1;13(1):41.

214. Simopoulos AP. The importance of the ratio of omega-6/omega-3 essential fatty acids. *Biomed Pharmacother.* 2002 Oct;56(8):365-379.

215. Simopoulos A: Omega-3 fatty acids in health and disease and in growth and development. *Am J Clin Nutr.* 1991;54:438-463.

216. Daley CA, Abbott A, Doyle PS, et al. A review of fatty acid profiles and antioxidant content in grass-fed and grain-fed beef. *Nutr J.* 2010;9:10. doi:10.1186/1475-2891-9-10.

217. Halvorsen BL. Blomhoff R.Determination of lipid oxidation products in vegetable oils and marine omega-3 supplements. *Food Nutr Res.* 2011;55. 10.3402/fnr.v55i0.5792

218. Grootveld M, Silwood CJ, Addis P, Health effects of oxidized heated oils. *Foodservice Research International.* 2001 october;13(1):41–55.

219. Santos CS, Cruz R. Cunha SC. Effect of cooking on olive oil quality attributes. *Food Research International.* [In Press, 2013]

220. Taubes, G. Which one will make you fat? Scientific American. September 2013. what-makes-you-fat-too-many-calories-or-the-wrong-carbohydrates. Accessed October 29, 2013.

221. Ebbeling CB, Swain JF, Feldman HA, et al. Effects of dietary composition on energy expenditure during weight-loss maintenance. *JAMA.* 2012;307:2627-2634.

222. Institute of Medicine. *Dietary reference intakes for water, potassium, sodium, chloride, and sulfate.* 1st ed. Washington, DC: The National Academies Press, 2004. http://www.iom.edu/Reports/2004/Dietary-Reference-Intakes-Water-Potassium-Sodium-Chloride-and-Sulfate. aspx. Accessed October 29, 2013.

223. He FJ, MacGregor GA. A comprehensive review of salt and health and current experience of worldwide salt reduction programmes. *J Hum Hypertens.* 2009;23:363-384.

224. Stein LJ, Cowart BJ, Beauchamp GK. The development of salty taste acceptance is related to dietary experience in human infants: a prospective study. *Am J Clin Nutr.* 2012 Jan;95(1):123-129.

225. Egan BM, Zhao Y, Axon RN. US trends in prevalence, awareness, treatment and control of hypertension, 1988-2008. *JAMA.* 2010;303(20):2043-2050.

226. Vasan RS, Beiser A, Seshadri S, et al. Residual lifetime risk for developing hypertension in middle-aged women and men: The Framingham Heart Study. *JAMA.* 2002;287:1003-1010.

References

227. John P. Forman, MD, MSc; Meir J. Stampfer, MD, DrPH; Gary C. Curhan, MD, ScD. Diet and Lifestyle Risk Factors Associated With Incident Hypertension in Women. *JAMA*. 2009;302(4):401-411.

228. Bibbins-Domingo K, Chertow GM, Coxson PG, et al. Projected effect of dietary salt reductions on future cardiovascular disease. *N Engl J Med*. 2010;362:590-599.

229. National Research Council. *Sodium Intake in Populations: Assessment of Evidence*. Washington, DC: The National Academies Press, 2013. Report brief. http://www.iom.edu/Reports/2013/Sodium-Intake-in-Populations-Assessment-of-Evidence/Report-Brief051413.aspx. Accessed October 29, 2013.

230. Turban S, Thompson CB, Parekh RS, Appel LJ. Effects of sodium intake and diet on racial differences in urinary potassium excretion: results from the Dietary Approaches to Stop Hypertension (DASH)-Sodium trial. *Am J Kidney Dis*. 2013;61:88-95.

231. Morbidity and Mortality Weekly Report. Sodium Intake Among Adults --- United States 2005–2006. *MMWR*. June 25, 2010; 59(24):737-768. http://www.cdc.gov/mmwr/preview/mmwrhtml/mm5924a4.htm?s_cid=mm5924a4_w. Accessed October 29, 2013.

232. National Cancer Institute. Applied Research Program. *Sources of Sodium Among the US Population, 2005-06*. National Cancer Institute. http://riskfactor.cancer.gov/diet/foodsources/sodium/. Accessed October 29, 2013.

233. Mattes RD, Donnelly D. Relative contributions of dietary sodium sources. *J Am Coll Nutr*. 1991;10:383-393.

234. Institute of Medicine. Consensus Report. *Strategies to Reduce Sodium Intake in the United States*. Released April 20, 2010. http://www.iom.edu/Reports/2010/Strategies-to-Reduce-Sodium-Intake-in-the-United-States.aspx. Accessed October 29, 2013.

235. Cobb LK, Appel LJ, Anderson CA. Strategies to Reduce Dietary Sodium Intake. *Curr Treat Options Cardiovasc Med*. 2012 August;14(4):425-434.

236. Adrogue HJ, Madias NE. Sodium and potassium in the pathogenesis of hypertension. *N Engl J Med*. 2007;356:1966-1978.

237. D'Elia L, Barba G, Cappuccio FP, et al. Potassium, stroke and cardiovascular disease. A meta-analysis of prospective studies. *J Am Coll Cardiol.* 2011;57:1210-1219.

238. Rebholz CM, Gu D, Chen J Physical activity reduces salt sensitivity of blood pressure: the Genetic Epidemiology Network of Salt Sensitivity Study. *Am J Epidemiol.* 2012 Oct 1;176(7):S106-S113. doi: 10.1093/aje/kws266.